Natural & Organic Healing

Your Ultimate Guide to Health & Wellness
2016

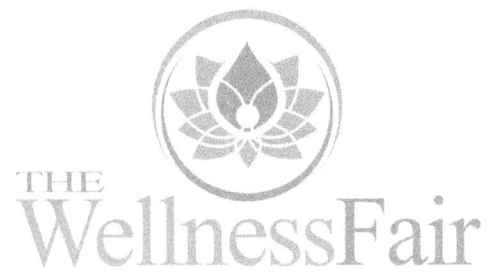

www.TheWellnessFair.org

organized by: Lucas J. Robak

Co-Authors From Wisconsin & Beyond

b

Contributing Wellpreneurs

Cindy L. Goodson
Lucas J. Robak
Nicole Isler
Sherry Brantley
Danielle LaRock
Diane Garrison, Ph.D.
Rich Perry
Deborah Crowe
David Fife
Dr. Matt Frahm
Heddy Keith
Keridak Silk
Allan Wich

"Sedentary people are apt to have sluggish minds.
A sluggish mind is apt to be reflected in flabbiness of body and in a
dullness of expression that invites no interest and gets none."
~ Rose Fitzgerald Kennedy ~

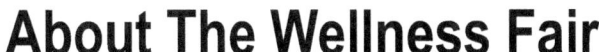

About The Wellness Fair

The Wellness Fair unites accredited wellness professionals with those who desire complete well-being. Our community naturally integrates the health of the whole body; physical, mental, emotional, and spiritual.

Online Wellness

Whether it's by attending our local trade fairs and speaking events or going online to consume the wisdom our community shares, you're bound to find that one golden nugget you need to improve your overall wellness.

There are various ways you can learn from our International qualified wellness professionals. You already started by picking up this book. Every November 1st, we release that years anthology book on Amazon. Mark your calendars because only in the month of November are all the volumes discounted for holiday gifts.

By going to our website, you'll also gather a great deal of information through our guest blog, *Thriving Naturally*. Every quarter we also release a new issue of our digital magazine, *Pathways 2 Wellness*. Finally, if you're really not the reading type, you're able to learn from practitioners from around the world on our podcast, *Healthy Conversations*.

Local Events

Attendees now have the ability to join our community to connect with service providers, learn a variety of health tips, and have their voice heard whenever it's convenient for them.

Our annual trade fairs consist of educational classes, workshops, and presentations to empower you to live a healthier lifestyle. To maintain the highest quality for you, all our presenters are chosen one month before the fair during our speakers conference called, *The Speakers Jam.*

Thousands of attendees are able to connect with hundreds of wellness practitioners all year. Visit our website and mark your calendars.

Getting Active

There are many ways you can get involved with our community:

1. Attend events as a wellness enthusiast
2. Consume our wisdom sharing materials
3. Be a vendor at a local trade fair nearest you
4. Once a vendor, you're able to be a speaker
5. Become a co-author in the next volume of this book series
6. Contribute to our guest blog
7. Contribute to our quarterly magazine
8. Be a guest on our podcast
9. Volunteer
10. Sponsor
11. Acquire a license to host events in your area

By partnering with us, you can leverage our community for an entire career; we'll train you how.

Does this seem like something you would be interested in?

Go to www.TheWellnessFair.org and sign up today.

Thank you!

Dedication

This book is dedicated to all those seeking a natural and healthy lifestyle. We hope you find that one golden nugget to improve your spiritual, mental, emotional, physical, or business well-being.

"In a disordered mind, as in a disordered body,
soundness of health is impossible."
~ Marcus Tullius Cicero ~

Table of Contents

Cindy L. Goodson, M.A., M.S., C.H.N.

Cindy Goodson refuses to let anything hold her life back. She's a doctoral candidate in health psychology with master's degrees in literature and fitness and human performance. She's a grandmother. She was once an R&B singer on the Billboard charts who still loves to perform any chance she gets. She has a passion for teaching others and has done so at the high school, college and community levels.

Cindy has a lot to live for, and thinks you do too. That's why her near-death experience with uterine fibroids drove her to take control of her health, healed her fibroids and begin to share her story for the benefit of others. Her first book, *Ladies Stop Thinking Start Shrinking: A 10 Step Guide to Shrinking Your Body and Your Fibroids Fast*, is based on her own journey of healing herself of debilitating fibroids through holistic nutrition.

Cindy has combined the knowledge gained from this journey along with all of her life lessons to launch *The Cindy G Project – A Health, Sassy & Wise Revolution*.

"To me, good health is more than just exercise and diet.
It's really a point of view and a mental attitude you have about yourself."
~ Albert Schweitzer ~

Houston, Texas, USA

Learn more by visiting www.cindylgoodson.com

Foreword

One of the biggest problems with our current healthcare system in America is that it is a badly broken misnomer, and is in reality, more of a disease-care system aimed at pushing pills and knives. Though quite an embarrassment, it is true, that the United States spends more money per capita on "healthcare" than any other country. Still, our nation is the sickest, the fattest, the unhappiest, and the most ignorant to the fact that healing power is right in our hands and all we have to do is tap into it.

Understanding the challenges that come with the ability to tap into our power of transformation, it is quite refreshing to know a book like the "Natural & Organic Healing: The Ultimate Guide to Health & Wellness" is available to guide us step-by-step on this ultimate healing journey. A Journey that for many, may seem out of reach because of the current state one may be experiencing at this time.

Furthermore, most are victims of a superimposed Western medical belief system that gives misleading information that shapes our perceptions around health and wellness from a Standard American Dietary perspective. The acronym for Standard American Diet is S.A.D., and sadly this system is the cause of what is ailing us, and it is not the cure.

Unfortunately, the medical and scientific research establishments, far from embrace these evidence-based findings, and go the extra mile to systematically dismiss and even suppress them. For that, I give praise to Lucas Robak and his team of collaborators in this excellent work.

When it comes to our personal life's curriculum involving our plan for shaping our psychology, our physiology, our productivity and our level of persuasion, most are inadequately equipped to master these major life areas and therefore, struggle at life-mastery.

As a health psychologist and certified holistic nutritionist, I deeply understand the importance of the work in these four areas. Likewise, I am astounded by how little most people (myself included, not too long ago) understand when it comes to something as simple as the power of food and the power of our perceptions around eating to live versus eating emotionally or eating because of our addictions. Not so simple, however, is being able to break free from the grip of addiction of the ill chemically laden foods that drive our culture right into the pit of sickness and disease, mentally physically, and spiritually.

After landing in critical ICU for the second time in the same year from iron deficiency anemia and requiring emergency blood transfusions, I knew I had to make a complete life changing transition to plant-based eating in order to save my life. The transfusions were necessary because of the debilitating symptoms of (9) large uterine fibroid tumors that had taken over my womb and left me hopelessly depressed, with no quality of life, and minutes from being lifeless.

I refused surgery because I wasn't going to be on the list with the other 600,000 hysterectomies being performed each year due to fibroids, and I decided to take the path of natural healing. After thousands of hours of research, and application, I am thoroughly convinced that most of those surgeries are unwarranted, and I will not be a statistic in that medical/big pharma business scandal.

Knowledge of holistic health and healing is powerful. Moreover, when implemented, it can change the trajectory of one's future in every way. It starts right here, with your health and your healing. I can sincerely say that if I did not have the type of information that is available in this guidebook and had I not surrounded myself with an amazing support system like Lucas Robak, and his team of experts, I would not be here today. I would have missed my calling to be sharing in this labor of love spreading the gospel of holistic health and healing. You too, have the power to *Design the Life You Desire to Live*, and *Live in The Body You Love to Love!*

*"My own prescription for health is less paperwork
and more running barefoot through the grass."*
~ Leslie Grimutter ~

Lucas J. Robak

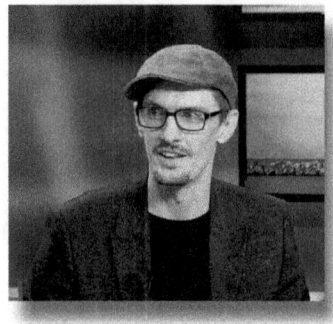

As a former pilot, wine maker, and teacher, Lucas J. Robak is a #1 bestselling author and a contributor to numerous publications like *Addicted 2 Success*, *Good Men Project*, and *Thrive Global*.

After publishing 75 people around the world for fun, he saw a need and is now considered to be the Entrepreneurs Publisher with *Authorpreneur Academy*.

A diagnosis of multiple sclerosis (MS) motivated Lucas to become a leader of *The Wellness Fair* by connecting qualified wellness professionals to those who desire a natural and healthy lifestyle.

This book series is a way for him to fulfill his purpose, "to help people become aware of their bodies natural ability to heal itself." Enjoy!

"Most people have no idea how good their body is designed to feel."
~ *Kevin Trudeau* ~

Milwaukee, Wisconsin, USA

Website: www.LucasRobak.com

Social Media:
- www.linkedin.com/in/LucasJRobak/
- www.facebook.com/LucasJRobak
- www.instagram.com/LucasJRobak

Enjoy growing as a person? Me too! Check out this list of my Top 150 Recommended Books (no email required) www.LucasRobak.com/150books

Introduction

"You can't connect the dots looking forward; you can only connect them looking backwards. So you have to trust that the dots will somehow connect in your future. You have to trust in something - your gut, destiny, life, karma, whatever. This approach has never let me down, and it has made all the difference in my life."
~ Steve Jobs ~

Imagine this! You're sitting alone in a hospital bed because you chose not to tell anyone you're checking yourself into one of their weekend suites.

What brought you to the Emergency Room that evening is one side of your body decided to stop working for a couple weeks; and it now hurts like hell.

Everyday you're exhausted the moment you wake up. Thinking is now a chore. Walking a straight line is near impossible, even using a walker is finally out of the question. Holding something in your hands, well, forget about that one, your left hand doesn't work anymore. Want to read something? Have someone read it to you instead because of how blurred your vision is. Make sure you clear your calendar when it's time to go to the bathroom, it could take an hour to start going and even longer to stop. Your short term memory is on strike, but only when it wants to be. To make sure life is even more interesting by creating embarrassing moments, remembering the names and faces of those you already know becomes questionable.

This was my life before a team of neurologists in the stroke unit at Froedtert Hospital in Milwaukee, WI handed me my life's purpose on a silver platter.

Hi! I'm Lucas J. Robak, the organizer of *The Wellness Fair* and the organizing author of this book series, *Natural & Organic Healing*.

I was gifted with the diagnosis of multiple sclerosis (MS) on May 30, 2014.

What is MS? I don't care what it is nor do I care about what it could possibly, might potentially do to me at some unforeseen point in the future. That knowledge is useless and pointless to me. I'm not a doctor, have never played one on T.V., and I didn't stay at a Holiday Inn Express last night. It's not my job to know anything about MS.

The only thing that matters is what's 100% in my control. How do I successfully live with one of the most debilitating neurological disorders known to mankind? The answer, this book and everything else I'm doing with my life!

The only challenge I've come across with developing this mentality is there are more than enough people out there who consistently force information on me which was never asked for. It's as if people purposefully want me to choose to become a hypochondriac so they can feel even worse for me. Don't make yourself out to be the victim due to my thinking. I'm not a victim of MS until I consciously choose to make that decision for myself.

Years leading up to that glorious moment at Froedtert, I was digging deep within myself to discover my purpose in life after attempting suicde in college. From experience, I knew it wasn't doing what society told me to do. Already did all that and it's not for me, hence the suicide attempt.

The beautiful Earl Nightingale tells me on a daily basis through his audiobook, *The Strangest Secret*, "The opposite of courage in our society is not cowardice... it is conformity." I spent a huge chunk of my life living like a conformed coward and it almost killed me.

Every now and then Art Williams pops in my life to say 'hi' through his 1987 speech, *Just Do It*. He loves reminding me, "... the only way not to be controversial is to be average and ordinary. Just call me anything but average and ordinary."

"If I want to be free, I've gotta be me. Not the me I think you think I should be.
Not the me I think my wife thinks I should I be. Not the me I think my kids think I
should be. But if I want to be free, I've gotta be.
So I'd better know who me is."
~ Bill Gove ~

I personally believe that conformity is a mental illness. The reason being is because when you do what your told, think what you're told to think, and act the way society demands you to act, you're not you - you're doing what the people in power dictate down to you instead; you're controlled by others.

The person who you're truly meant to be is dying inside because you want society to look upon as "one of us." Well, thankfully, I'm not you, I'm me! And if I wanna be free, I've gotta be me!

Once I started down the path of "being me," that's when everything started to come together ... and fall apart.

What fell apart were most of my prior relationships, we were no longer thinking and functioning on the same frequency. We either naturally drifted away from each other, or I purposefully burnt the bridge to end that negative part of my life.

What came together, was me! Through books, videos, seminars, conferences, writing with a pen on paper, and a lot of status quo resistance, I deliberately transformed my life into what I consciously mapped out.

Before continuing, I'd like to make clear that I'm not saying suicide or chronic illnesses are a positive thing, they're not. What I've intentionally reprogrammed myself to do is to seek out the positives buried within the negatives; make this simple decision and you can easily do it too.

If I never attempted sucide, I never would have started down the path of personal development. I never would have came to realize first-hand how powerful we all are. Without medication, and without therapy, I thought myself out of depression and into the life you're seeing today. I chose to do it this way because I figured if one can think themselves into suicide, just imagine the possibilities of what you can think yourself into on the positive end of the spectrum.

Now onto my glorious MS, the real reason you have this book in your hands.

For over a decade I trained myself to ignore my body because I equated it to be like my car, if you keep driving, that "clunk" will fix itself ... and it does every time. In 2014 I came to realize that when my body "fixed itself," that was just an active lesion in my brain or spine dying off.

I'm sure you're somewhat the same too. Every time your body tries to tell you something, do you actually listen and do something about it or just keep going about your life like I did?

Metaphorically speaking, my body was beating the hell out of me and I took like a champ - I thought everyone experienced this. I didn't want to be one of those people who go to the ER just because I blew my nose. By the way, due to MS, I'm always the healthiest person in every room because my immune system is stronger than it should be. What does "blowing your nose" even mean? Can't remember the last time that happened to me. Jealous of my MS yet?

While sitting in the hospital bed for three days, once I was done working, I found time to start researching MS. After reading the first sentence in my first search I instantly learned to stop looking up MS. Instead, I started researching how to successfully live with a chronic illness.

Guess what I found? Exactly what we all should be doing in the first place!

Natural, organic, Eastern medicine … preventative care! There's no need to swallow a bunch of pills if you actually take care of yourself, right?

Personally, I believe the only reason this isn't mainstream yet is because there isn't billions of dollars to be made and no patents can be filed. The pharmaceutical companies, lobbyists, politicians, FDA officials, hospitals, and nonprofits stand to lose hundreds of billions of dollars every year once the world wakes up to natural health and their bodies innate ability to heal itself without doing hardcore drugs. Western medicine would cease to exist outside the ER and diagnostics.

This is my goal, my purpose in life, my obligation to the world!

Without going to the Lobbyist store and making an expensive purchase to legally own the decisions of a few politicians and numerous FDA officials, we can achieve this goal of perfect health by simply gaining the knowledge provided within this book series.

My obligation in life: "to help the world become aware of their bodies natural ability to heal itself." And I'm not going to be the one delivering the message, nor the one working one-on-one with people; let's leave that to the professionals in this book series.

> *"The best way to predict the future is to create it."*
> *~ Abraham Lincoln ~*

To achieve my purpose in life, I'm the back seat driver. Instead of me striving to be the next big thing in the wellness world; I work with wellpreneurs to help them effectively reach more people.

Even though I have my master practitioner certification in Neuro-Linguistic Programming (NLP), master hypnotherapist certification, and Reiki Level II certification; instead of me working with you directly pertaining to your health goals, I'm now working with wellness professionals for them to gain more visibility and credibility in the marketplace so you can find them easier.

Do you like what you've read from a particular co-author?

Reach out and hire them - they'd do a far better job with you than I ever could! I'm simply just a community organizer and entrepreneur publisher. The co-authors are the ones who'll be there to change your life, it's no longer me.

- Thankfully, I attempted suicide.
- Thankfully, I developed and become aware of MS.
- Thankfully, I chose to create the mentality I did to seek the positives when society wants you to choose victimhood instead.

Because of all this, *The Wellness Fair* exists. Because of all this, you're reading a wonderful book filled with imperative information, that once converted to knowledge through implementation, could revolutionize your entire well-being.

Enjoy this book, read the other books within the *Natural & Organic Healing* series, connect with all the contributing authors, and at some point, I'll be seeing you at our next wellness event!

With love and appreciation,

Lucas J. Robak

Community Organizer
www.TheWellnessFair.org/Lucas

Lucas J. Robak

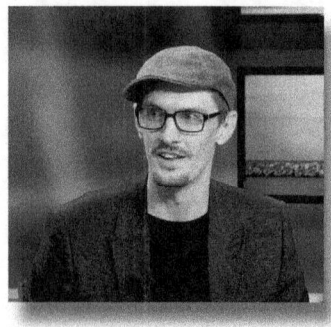

As a former pilot, wine maker, and teacher, Lucas J. Robak is a #1 bestselling author and a contributor to numerous publications like *Addicted 2 Success*, *Good Men Project*, and *Thrive Global*.

After publishing 75 people around the world for fun, he saw a need and is now considered to be the Entrepreneurs Publisher with *Authorpreneur Academy*.

A diagnosis of multiple sclerosis (MS) motivated Lucas to become a leader of *The Wellness Fair* by connecting qualified wellness professionals to those who desire a natural and healthy lifestyle.

This book series is a way for him to fulfill his purpose, "to help people become aware of their bodies natural ability to heal itself." Enjoy!

"Most people have no idea how good their body is designed to feel."
~ *Kevin Trudeau* ~

Milwaukee, Wisconsin, USA

Website: www.LucasRobak.com

Social Media:
- www.linkedin.com/in/LucasJRobak/
- www.facebook.com/LucasJRobak
- www.instagram.com/LucasJRobak

Enjoy growing as a person? Me too! Check out this list of my Top 150 Recommended Books (no email required) www.LucasRobak.com/150books

Successfully Live with a
Chronic Illness

On a monthly basis very smart people in white coats holding clipboards tell me I have multiple sclerosis (MS). Since being diagnosed with one of the most debilitating neurological disorders; I've learned a lot of information, met many phenomenal people both in-person and online, been interviewed multiple times, received invitations to speak and do group coaching, became more organized, feel healthier than ever, and raised the bar on all of my goals. Thank you MS!

"Things work out best for those who make the best of the way things work out."
~ John Wooden ~

Once my life purpose was handed to me on a silver platter, I did what anyone would do in that situation, looked up the foreign word I was just diagnosed with. What a stupid mistake that was! Why do we purposefully make matters worse when we can easily choose the better action?

After reading the first sentence in Wikipedia, I chose not to give a damn about this auto-immune/neurological disorder. People way smarter than I'll ever be who dedicated their lives to researching and treating MS have a reason to learn about it, not me. How is my life and health going to get better knowing that I can forget what my loved ones look like while they're changing my diaper because my limbs forgot how to communicate with my brain? And that is all before breakfast.

Schoolhouse Rock needs to apologize to the world for lying to us all, "Knowledge is NOT power!" Knowledge is simply perceived power. Action and action alone is where your true power lies. So, with the knowledge of knowing I can poop myself, forget what my family looks like, have minimal use of my limbs, more susceptible to depression, unable to read, hear noises that aren't there, read words that weren't written, experience spasticity, forget what I'm doing, have intense insomnia with disabling fatigue; what action can I take with this useless knowledge from hell?

The only thing I can come up with is that I now have the knowledge and ability to turn myself into a crippled victim.

I am the creator of my life. I am the only one who is responsible for my health, wealth, and personal fulfillment. My thoughts, decisions, and actions created my MS. No more researching what the illness is, that's my doctor's job. My job is to take care of myself so that I can achieve all my outlandish goals which make other people nervous. I can't be a starting NFL quarterback if I choose to think myself into becoming a quadriplegic.

After reading that one Wikipedia sentence, it was an easy choice to switch gears and research "How to Successfully Live with Multiple Sclerosis."

Weeks of this research and hundreds of hours of personal development seminars, I think I unofficially cracked the code into living a healthy life with a chronic illness. Before I begin, I've been advised to tell you I'm not a medical professional, I have no academic letters before or after my name, never even applied to graduate school, I have not been published in any medical journals, couldn't find one sentence in Grey's Anatomy I could understand, and still ask my doctors to talk to me like a child. Don't take medical advice from me, legally speaking!

There are nine techniques which are easy to implement and simple to follow. The hardest part is actually doing them habitually. Books are knowledge. That's that, nothing more. It's up to you to act on what you decide to act on.

With these nine simple tips, you could begin healing your physical, emotional, mental, and spiritual bodies in a more natural and holistic way.

1) Set Small Goals

> *"The best way to predict the future is to create it."*
> *~ Abraham Lincoln ~*

Focus on an outcome which you're passionate about the result. Dr. Patrick Hill and Dr. Nicholas Turiano "proved" that living a purposeful life promotes a happier, healthier, longer, and more fulfilling life. Purpose comes from our passions and is produced through acting on meaningful goals.

I can give you a list of my goals and most of them you wouldn't want to do. Your passions, purpose, and desires are yours. Be proud of who you are and pursue a life worth bragging about. Whatever you dream of is perfect for you!

Whether it's in the area of health, relationships, career, finances, school, environment, family, personal development, spiritual growth, etc. set one tiny little goal to achieve each day, week, month, quarter, and/or year. Start with just one, and go from there.

2) Self-Talk

"If you keep saying things are going to be bad,
you have a chance of being a prophet."
~ Isaac Singer ~

Affirmations are the best way to reprogram your subconscious mind into operating the way you direct it to. Since our subconscious runs 90-95% of our daily lives, reprogramming it is essential to achieve anything we've never done before. Through our parents, teachers, coaches, friends, family, etc. our subconscious has been programmed to operate a certain way.

If you watch the news, you need a massive overhaul of your subconscious.

When choosing an affirmation, make sure everything is stated in the positive-present-tense. Include a feeling which you'll experience once achieving this result along with an action word ending in -ing. Start it with either "I am…", "I have…", or "I do…" to begin thinking you already have it. That's the key, this is where the magic happens.

Write this down and carry it with you everywhere you go.

Repeat the affirmation thousands of times a day for 90 days. Within time you'll notice your thoughts, decisions, and actions changing to align your external world with your internal beliefs. Why think yourself into the morgue when you can think yourself into maximum achievement?

3) Exercise

"Those who think they have no time for exercise
will sooner or later have to find time for illness."
~ Edward Stanley ~

Who cares if you're not in the VIP Chronic Illness Club, everyone should exercise at minimum 10-30 minutes every day.

I was a lab rat at Marquette University's study with Dr. Alex Ng to verify that ballroom dancing has benefits for those with MS. It does!

It gets your heart rate up and keeps you moving instead of watching the "boob-tube" all day on an overly comfortable Lay-Z-Boy.

There are so many ways to exercise. Go for a walk, do yoga, take a dance class, lift weights, climb stairs, do t'ai chi, move some furniture, do the dishes, golf, rake leaves...anything to get you moving around and your blood flowing.

If you can't physically exercise because of your progressive disease, Erin M. Shackell and Lionel G. Standing at Bishop's University "proved" how incredible our thoughts are. Just by visualizing working out, study subjects increased their strength by 24%.

4) Diet

> "The food you eat can be either the safest and most powerful form of medicine
> or the slowest form of poison."
> ~ Ann Wigmore ~

With all the chemicals and modifications to our food, it's no surprise that we have more health problems than corporations with politicians on payroll.

After a lot of research, asking questions in support groups, talking with real medical professionals, I found multiple diet tips to begin living a healthier life with food.

Stay away from: gluten, dairy, sugar, legumes/beans, pork, and red meat. Instead of using butter, use coconut oil. Instead of heating something up in the microwave, smash it with a sledge hammer. A friend once told me that instead of drinking Diet Coke, I should just shoot myself. After reading the research on aspartame, I agree with her extreme metaphor, I'm slowly killing myself by drinking it.

For MS, the diets that are recommended are SWANK, Paleo, Wahl's Protocol, alkaline, and the Blood Type Diet. Each one has many case studies "proving" that it works. When it comes to food, get to know your body as to which food and diets work best for you. You may find nothing here works...cool beans, keep looking!

5) Vitamins

"I take a multivitamin, vitamin D and omega-3 oils every day,
and if I'm stressed or run down, I bulk up on vitamin C and zinc."
~ L'Wren Scott ~

When we cook our food, we lose nutrients. When we microwave it, might as well eat dirt. Raw vegetables have the most nutrients, but for me, my pizza doesn't have all the fruit and vegetables I need in a daily serving; this is where supplements come in.

When I first met with my neurologist, he gave me a pamphlet of "all things Eastern" to improve health. In this, he suggested many vitamins and minerals for those with a MS. Looking at his material, I wondered why schools chose not to add this to the curriculum since it's information for everyone.

Out of what I learned, we all can focus on vitamin D and omega-3. In my unprofessional opinion, these are the two most important vitamins to take. Whether or not you're the healthiest one in the room, start taking these. Low vitamin-D levels can create MS. If you're like me, vitamin-D can help to ward off flare ups. Omega-3 is great for the brain. Your brain controls everything. Common sense says to take omega-3 fish oil.

6) Physiology

"Smile if it kills you. The physiology of smiling diffuses a lot of anger and angst.
It makes your body and soul feel better."
~ Tom Peters ~

Our body posture not only projects our energy to the world, it has a direct impact on our internal well-being.

How can you feel good about yourself when you slouch all the time? How will your confidence shine when your chin is angled down? What benefits can you lie to yourself about receiving by frowning most of the time?

I personally have experienced the profound impact of physiology in my health. Sit up straight, shoulder blades are closer together rather than positioned slightly forward, chin angled slightly up, smile, feet just a little wider than shoulder width apart, elbows bent with hands clasped above the naval, eyes above the horizon, inhaling through the nose while exhaling through the mouth, hips forward, and keep the knees slightly bent. This can happen while sitting too!

7) Reading

> *"Reading is to the mind what exercise is to the body."*
> *~ Joseph Addison ~*

The information we indulge in creates the energy we carry with us throughout the day. My spiritual health was garbage when I use to read the news and what the president plans on doing next.

Learning about the Milwaukee ghetto isn't something that is going to allow me to easily project out positive energy.

To me, "Spiritual Health" is energy. The thoughts we have can come from the material we read. Quantum physics proves beyond a reasonable doubt that everything is energy. Our thoughts project out certain frequencies which repel and attract events and people into our lives.

My entire world changed when I chose to start reading self-help, self-empowerment, self-improvement, personal development, and success books. Because of this shift in genres, my spiritual energy shifted and the universe did exactly what it has been doing for eons.

After destroying your microwave, celebrate by doing the same to your TV set.

8) Pendulum

> *"The pendulum of the mind alternates between sense*
> *and nonsense, not between right and wrong."*
> *~ Carl Jung ~*

You now have a direct line of communication to the most powerful force in the universe. Communicate directly with the subconscious mind and produce immediate results. Through this technique, we play 20 questions with our minute muscle movements.

Put something with weight at the end of a string and you have yourself a pendulum. Mine has a key ring big enough for my index finger to fit in with a gemstone at the end of a chain.

While standing up, I put my finger in the key ring and allow the pendulum to freely dangle. Keeping my arm/elbow off my body, I look down to see which way the stone swings.

Direct your questioning to what decisions and actions you should take. This is not fortune telling. Since our subconscious knows everything, make sure you thank it for the answers received by following through with your insight.

9) Eastern Medicine

"Eastern medicine is not about curing sickness. It's about keeping you well."
~ Tim Daly ~

What an incredible way of life. Eastern medicine has been around for thousands of years with little change. Western medicine changes constantly. Eastern promotes healing and wellness. Western is great for ER, diagnosing, and covering up the problem.

When is covering up the problem okay? I receive a Tysabri infusion once a month. It's not fixing it. It's covering it up while risking my organs, and actually, my life. I'll continue this monthly ritual until my body rejects it.

Since my MS discovery and becoming the organizer of WIHHE, I learned so many "secrets". Find what works for you:

Meditation, floating, acupuncture, acupressure, massages, chiropractic, yoga, t'ai chi, Qigong, Feng Shui, Huna, reiki, essential oils, psychology, vitamins, herbs, and minerals, numerology, astrology, shiatsu, nutritional counseling, art/light/color/sound/music/vibrational/aroma therpay, energy/spiritual healing, hypnotherapy, NLP, and much, much more.

It's exciting to learn this is becoming more mainstream. Even Western science is starting to catch up to the ancient Eastern beliefs. When will our society?

*****

"It does not matter how slowly you go
as long as you do not stop."
~ Confucius ~

I'm not good at most of this. I forget to do it every day. I've known this information for nearly a decade and my health is still a work in progress, always will be.

Hopefully you found at least half of a sentence you want to experiment with to see if it's right for you. What works for one person may not work for you. That's what makes life so fun. Test, learn from what happened, change things if you need to, then test again, repeat. You'll find what works best for your body as long as you don't stop.

When pursuing better health or any desired outcome, nothing worthwhile is going to happen within 30 days. Sometimes it may take decades. Keep doing what is most right for you at that moment in time. Refer back to this book and the other chapters to find that spark of motivation you need to keep going.

It took me nearly four years of failing to learn how to write and publish books efficiently and effectively. I believed I could do it, I had the desire to do it, so I did it, period! I don't care what my mom says, I'm not special! You have the ability to choose to do something and then do what it takes to achieve it. The only thing stopping you from optimal health is you.

For the next 90 days, no matter what room you're in, say to yourself, "I'm the healthiest person in this room." Since we already have a ton of false beliefs about the world around us, why not believe that? I believe it!

*****

"Anything I can do you can do better.
It's a matter of belief backed by desire."
~ Lucas J. Robak ~

"What the mind can conceive and believe,
the mind can achieve."
~ Napoleon Hill ~

Nicole Isler

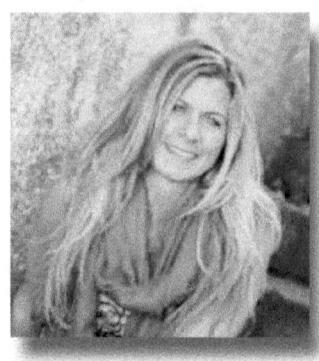

Nicole M. Isler is a Coach for Sensitive Souls. She helps highly sensitive people go from feeling flawed and broken to feeling confident and free, by embracing their gift of sensitivity as their superpower.

She is the CEO of Big Dream Awakening, forthcoming author of *Go With Your Gut*, host of *Positivity Party Radio* and creator of *The Navigator*, a holistic methodology that teaches HSP to navigate their emotions so they can thrive and be happy.

The Sensitive Souls Nicole has worked with have gone on to become professional artists, healers, published authors, successful entrepreneurs, empowered parents and superheros.

The secret of health for both mind and body is not to mourn for the past,
not to worry about the future, or not to anticipate troubles,
but to live in the present moment wisely and earnestly.
~ Buddha ~

Waukesha, Wisconsin, USA

Website: http://bigdreamawakening.com

Social Media:
- www.facebook.com/bigdreamawakening/

Take the next step. Connect with Nicole for a Sensitivity Scan:
http://bit.ly/FreeSensitivtyScan

Sensitivity or Superpower

Have you ever been told you're "too sensitive"?
Does it make you feel like you have to be on guard with your emotions?

I know how you feel. I felt the same way but I found a way to navigate through the frustration, isolation, and discomfort.

I want you to know there is a way out, you can be happy, and you can use your sensitivity in a way that it becomes your superpower.

As long as I can remember, my hyper-sensitivity has been a running theme in my life. It held me back from trying new things, expressing my feelings and being successful.

People in my life would say things like…

- "Don't be so sensitive"
- "Don't take everything so personal"
- "Stop being so emotional"

Every time this would happen, I would own it. It must be me. I was being too sensitive again.

I tried to hide it, act like nothing bothered me so people would leave me alone. My feelings became insignificant because someone determined I was 'overthinking' something and I believed them.

Does any of this remind you of yourself — or someone close to you? If so, you're not crazy or weak or "too sensitive." You are not broken and there is definitely nothing wrong with you.

You are a sensitive soul, a Highly Sensitive Person. (HSP) And it's not a bad thing. You can learn to use your sensitivity, as your superpower.

I'm here to tell you…

Be who you are, make no apologies.

We sensitive types live in a world of people who don't necessarily understand or appreciate our strong feelings. They just don't get it. And for some reason, we translate that to "there must be something wrong with me".

When actually, your sensitivity is what's absolutely right about you.

When you are told "you're too sensitive", it eats away at your self-esteem, you start to feel abnormal. Self-doubt sets in and you take a step back from living the life you truly want.

Your dreams slip away bit by bit.

Sensitive Souls are greatly misunderstood and hugely undervalued. They are looked down upon for being a deep feeling person.

Hypersensitivity, often mislabeled as shyness, is generally treated as a character flaw. Being treated this way can leave you feeling like an outcast in society, your workplace or even your own family gatherings.

Due to your feelings of frustration, you might experience angry outbursts, anxiety, and depression and have a deep desire to just 'be normal'.

You're not alone if that resonates and sadly the numbers are adding up. There are currently 40 million adults affected by anxiety disorders and 14.8 by depression in the United States alone.

Those are staggering statistics. Too many people are going through life feeling broken, out of control, isolated and in many cases, medicated.

It doesn't have to be that way.

What if instead, I told you that you are gifted? That's right, I said gifted.

Being highly sensitive is not a flaw, it's not just part of your genetic make-up, it's your genius make-up. It's your superpower.

However, until you fully understand it, it will feel like a curse, not the blessing it was meant to be.

Most of the people around you have no idea what it feels like to be you. Only 15-20% of the population has the ability to feel and sense energy the way you do.

While this trait is not a new discovery, it has not been honored in the way it should be. It has been mislabeled as something bad.

I'm here to tell you times are changing. Sensitives are gaining respect and honor and there's science to back it up.

A study by Stony Brook University psychologists found your brain as an HSP works a little differently than others. You're more aware of your surroundings, you process information more thoroughly and you have the ability to pick up on other people's emotional cues as if they are your own.

When you're in balance or in alignment, this works in your favor, as a gift, leading you to your best life as your best self.

Your relationships flourish, you feel a deeper connection with those around you and build rapport very quickly. People enjoy being around you because you seem to 'get them', they're drawn to you for your insight and creative perspectives.

You feel energized and strong, vitality is plentiful. You allow life to unfold for you, trusting your inner guidance to help you make decisions.

However, when you're out of alignment, you may feel out of sorts, like you're not right, confused, overthinking, weighed down and far from the life you dream of living.

You start to isolate, feeling no one seems to 'get you'. You worry what other people think of you. You start projects but never seem to finish them. You feel overwhelmed.

This drains you, you feel off. You start to lose sight of possibilities and feel like a failure.

Being in balance is not as much about being in balance as it is noticing when you're out of balance. There are signs and symptoms to help you recognize when you need to adjust.

Using your sensitivity as your superpower comes down to having the right mindset and continuously reading your own energy to notice when you're out of alignment.

This is your time. Embrace your gift of sensitivity. You can flourish as an HSP. The best thing you can do is check in with your feelings, notice what you notice.

Here's are 5 HSP qualities when you're in alignment and symptoms to watch for if you drift.

1) **In alignment:** You process information more thoroughly. You are able to process material at deeper levels with long periods of focus and concentration. This can lead to wonderful creations, inventions, and ideas. Known as an 'out of the box' thinker you have the ability to see things from endless directions creating new perspectives when others may see only limited approaches.

- **Out of alignment:** Over-analyze everything down a destructive path until your mind is racing toward dead ends. This snowballs, draining energy and cluttering your mind. When group brainstorming and team projects are not productive, creative, fun or are too rigid, you may feel stifled and limited resulting in withdrawal, disengagement, and even resentment.

2) **In alignment:** You have an especially strong empathetic response to emotional cues from others. Greatest social fulfillment tends to come from close relationships, and this is where you are able to shine. You have the ability to feel what others feel, like emotional x-ray vision. You are most likely the go-to person when it comes to helping others feel better or feel understood. You build rapport with ease and connect with others quickly, meeting someone where they're at emotionally without the other person having to explain what they feel.

- **Out of alignment:** Tend not to share openly with just anyone, will not share with someone you sense negativity from. In the workplace, if you feel forced to "play office politics" you may rebel when pushed. Colleagues or acquaintances may not understand this behavior and may label you as aloof, arrogant or cold. Your energy hardens as a result of over-protection, like a shell, closing off others even more. Emotions can feel cluttered, hard to separate what is self and what is others. You may put up a wall if hurt in the past. If self-esteem is low (because society doesn't view the HSP traits as ideal), you may fall in love with someone your inferior. The tendency to overextend to others, creating feelings of resentment and overwhelm, compensate by withdrawing or isolating to release the pressure. It's easy for an untrained sensitive to take in everyone else's stuff and feel weighed down or confused as to what to do with it. There's no separation between what is self and what is others.

3) In alignment: You can pick up on subtleties that others overlook like things in the air, temperature changes, lights, fabrics, scents, and odors. Highly skilled at tasks that involve observing minor differences. Can see the unseen, feel the vibe and adapt or adjust accordingly. Sensitives make great scientists, detectives, caretakers, animal healers, parents, teachers, energy workers, coaches, and psychologists.

- **Out of alignment:** If overstimulated, you feel overwhelmed, frantic or anxious. Tend to shut down, pull away. Cannot 'think straight', process ideas or organize details mentally. Your mind will only focus on the unwanted sensory stimulation like loud noise, unpleasant odor, etc. May feel out of control, cramped or too much pressure. Racing thoughts become over focused on the negative details escalating anxiety.

4) In alignment: You have an active imagination. Your creative mind is always running and ideas can spark at any moment. This gives you a strong appreciation for the fine details of art and music because you can feel the meaning behind the creation. You live a more vivid and inspired life filled with deep meaning, beauty, and ability to create peaceful environments with natural/earth elements that are visually soothing.

- **Out of alignment:** Feelings of too many ideas and not enough time. Inspiration has no traction, unfinished projects – always starting, never completing. May have a lot of interests but there's no feeling of sense or order, leaving you feeling scattered and confused. Your environment can become cluttered, you feel overwhelmed, cramped, feelings of defeat and failure take over zapping your inspiration.

5) In alignment: You are natural born entrepreneur. Conscientious about planning and research, you excel at being self-employed. You love to control the many aspects of your life and business, the hours, stimulation, kinds of people you deal with and product/services you offer. This keeps you living inspired. Unlike many first-time entrepreneurs, you balance risk with making an impact. Can see the 'bigger picture', and live to make the world a better place through your service to others. Because connection comes easily to you, you see the world as one and feel happiest when making a difference and using your gifts.

- **Out of balance:** You worry excessively and unnecessarily, thinking too deeply on projects, wanting it to be perfect but always feeling it's flawed. May be inclined to work unthinkable hours to accomplish the big goal. Sacrifice self-care for productive hours, grinding down energy to burn-out levels. May lose interest if the creative mind works faster than the progress of the project.

5 tips to thrive and not slip off out of alignment:

1) **Plenty of playtime.** That means doing nothing, or doing something that requires no thinking energy. Examples might be sitting outside, spending time with your pet or favorite friend, watching a funny or favorite movie, cleaning, gardening...whatever you don't have to "figure anything out" to do. It's really for no other reason than to have fun.

2) **Be selective about your relationships.** Spend time with people who 'get you', who are super easy to be around. This makes conversation easier, it also generates energy for you. You feel understood and safe to open up and share about yourself as much as listen and help them. It's a give-give type of relationship.

3) **Get very clear about who you are.** Establish your independence and a strong sense of self and identity. Without everything in your life, who are you? If you can clearly and confidently answer that question, you'll feel centered and solid no matter what changes come your way.

4) **Plenty of alone time.** It's a must, even if non-HSP don't understand. Without this time, you cannot reach your full potential. Alone time is how you declutter emotionally and settle energetically, how you get back to self.

5) **Make self-care a priority.** It's imperative to care for your emotional, mental, physical and spiritual needs. Be sure to include daily actions and activities that fill each of these containers. Examples spend time in nature, massage, exercise, deep breathing, organic and whole foods, sleep, journaling, meditation, etc.

Bonus tip: Fully accept and embrace that being highly sensitive is your gift and your superpower. It makes you special and gives you the ability to help others in a meaningful way.

Your specialized, innate skills as a Highly Sensitive Person whether in business or personal settings can help you thrive and succeed. The more you develop, the stronger your superpower becomes, the more you shine, the happier you feel.

You can learn to navigate your feelings and use your emotions. You can be yourself 100%, a Sensitive Soul. You can be your own Superhero.

*"If you want to be happy, set a goal that commands your thoughts,
liberates your energy and inspires your hopes."*
~ Andrew Carnegie ~

Sherry Brantley

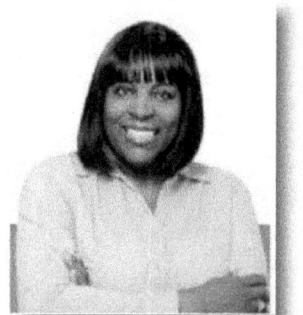

Sherry Brantley is the author of *STEPP-Start To Exercise Personal Power—How To Create Positive Change In Your Life*!

Sherry is a Certified Life Coach and Certified Professional Coach specializing in the areas of Goal-Setting and Goal Attaining!

She is a dynamic speaker and trainer. Whether writing books related to personal growth, poetry books or her award-winning fictional trilogy of work entitled *Best of Friends*, Sherry incorporates thought-provoking concepts which readers are able to connect to in order to increase their understanding of their own Spiritual Growth, to determine what they'd like to achieve in life!

"All successful people have a goal. No one can get anywhere unless he knows where he wants to go and what he wants to be or do."
~ Norman Vincent Peale ~

Scottsdale, Arizona, USA

Website: www.sherrybrantley.com

Social Media:
  • www.facebook.com/STEPP-745988562211755/

Get Your Free 'Goal-Getting' Coaching Session!
Send request to: yourdesiredlife@aol.com

Mistakes Most People Make When Setting Goals

Goals. What a wonderful tool we get to use in order to assist us in making our dreams come true! Goals help us to shape our destiny, create our future, and begin to experience the life we've always envisioned for ourselves.

Achieving our goals involves making sacrifices along the way, contrary to popular belief it's not a perquisite nor a requirement that you endure a long, uphill battle, neglect all other areas of your life, or that you must desert family and friends leaving you feeling 'all alone' as you pursue your dream. You'll discover it can be a lot simpler to achieve your goals rather they be large or small, once you have the proper tools to assist you.

Were you aware that studies indicate anywhere from 93% to 97% of the population do not achieve their goals? Do you fantasize about the type of life you would have if you'd completed your goals? Has your 'Bucket List,' become your 'I'll just 'shuck it' list?

I'll give you some easy techniques to jump clear over the hurdles that may have stopped you before. Once you begin to utilize this information on a consistent basis, you too, shall begin to join the ranks of those of us that are able to move beyond goal-setting—to Goal-Getting!

Goals, vision boards, bucket lists; no matter how you label them, they all boil down to one thing: People who are looking to move beyond their fears or prior protestations so they may begin to achieve their goals.

Many of us see our goals as 'someday,' or just before we get to the 'after-life.' You know what I mean: After the kids are grown; and then it's after the kids are actually gone, after I get the promotion, come back from vacation, or finish school. For some, goals are referred to as 'lifetime goals,' which gives the impression that they have a 'lifetime to achieve them,' or they're referred to as a 'bucket list' meaning they only need to focus on them prior to 'kicking the bucket.' Goals are placed on the back burner while the years of your life roll by. Goals don't just happen 'someday when you least expect them,' nor will your goals 'jump up and surprise you out of the blue without any input from you.'

While Vision Boards and affirmations are a great start towards beginning to realize your dreams, they are just that—a start. Focus and action will be the fuel that propels you to achieve your goals. Are YOU ready to go from 'Goal-Setting to Goal-Getting?'

The first mistake most people make when setting goals is they're focused on their goal being 'Too Big.' Stephen Covey stated to 'Begin with the end in mind,' which is great advice. However, too many people conjure up the image of that 'big picture' and while they are excited about that end goal, they fail to realize that it is just that—the end goal.

When you're focused on the 'Big Picture,' your mind also focuses on the big questions: The 'how,' the 'when' and the 'who will help along the way?' Not being able to answer these questions at this early stage of goal-setting makes people become paralyzed of the big picture and afraid of the enormity of it. You begin to doubt your dream and therefore, yourself. You wonder if you're deserving of such a lofty goal. Soon, you're relegating your mind to the idea that the goal was too much for you to achieve and you simply resign yourself to living your dreams— only in your mind.

A way to combat this goal-killer is to keep in mind the words of Martin L. King Jr., who stated, 'You don't have to see the entire staircase in order to take the first step.' If you're one of the many people who tend to get stuck at the idea of your big picture; if your goals seem too big to accomplish or too far down the road for you to take the first step, focus only on the steps that are right there in front of you. Not the entire staircase or the end goal. You do this by dividing your bigger goal into 'bite-sized chews,' so that you're not 'biting off more than you can chew.' You're then able to complete those smaller steps that are manageable for you at each leg of your progress. This allows you to experience success early on which fuels you to maintain your spark of enthusiasm as you work towards your ultimate goal.

The mantra to remember the 'Too Big' rule is: 'Bite-sized chews are right for you!'

As we can all attest, people have become accustomed to 'multi-tasking' and unfortunately, have carried that mentality to their goal-setting regimen. This causes many people to attempt to focus on too many projects at once while not doing any of them with any modicum of success. Therefore, the second common mistake most people make when setting their goals is focusing on trying to achieve 'Too Many' goals at once. We are able to focus on two to three major things at a time—for a short or 'temporary' period of time. However, when we try to give all of our energy and efforts to a vast array of projects over an extended period of time, we become the proverbial 'Jack of all trades—and master of none.' Our goals begin to slip away one by one.

We have all either witnessed this with others or we've been guilty of committing this error in our own lives. You know the scenario: It's the end of the year and the beginning of a New. Everyone's excited about really sticking with their New Year's resolution. Someone runs up to you and exclaims, "Sherry, I'm going to go back to school, finish my degree, join a gym, lose weight and find my soul-mate—all within the next 90 days!" Well, the bulk of New Year's resolutions never make it past the third week of January.

Before January ends, the resolutions have petered out, people realize they can't maintain such a frenetic pace of all of their lofty New Year plans without suffering physically, mentally, and depending on some of their goals, even financially. They begin to lose hope, see themselves as failures, begin beating themselves up mentally for their shortcomings and resign themselves to wait another entire year before repeating the same routine. Never mind that there are still eleven months of the year that can be utilized and mapped out for success. Their focus was on it being a 'New year and a new 'me,' and once the year has begun with little or no success, they feel that ship has left the harbor and sailed.

An easy fix to avoid this common mistake is to reflect on what you'd really like to achieve for the entire year—and then, piggy-backing from the first error I spoke of where goals seemed too big, divide your goals into quarterly goals. This means choosing only two or three of your goals to focus on at a time, rather than the goals you've mapped out for the entire year. This allows feasible time-frames within each of the quarterly 90-day periods to complete each of your goals without becoming too stressed or feelings of being overwhelmed.

Imagine focusing on just a few goals and giving them your undivided attention for 90-days. You'll be amazed at what that will do for you. You'll reach milestones you had not been able to complete before.

A great technique to add to this 'Too Many' error is to focus on 'like goals' to complete tasks in one goal set that overlaps into the other. For example; if your goal is to eat healthily and to lose weight, these would can be achieved in the same quarter.

As you begin to consciously choose your foods and incorporate a regimen of 'moving your body more,' and since your goals now go hand in hand, you're able to give your attention to these two goals without feeling it's too much of a stretch.

'Grouping like goals' together allows you to focus your attention properly on moving forward in two separate areas while achieving them both at the same time!

The mantra to remember the 'Too Many' rule is: Too many goals leads to feelings of despair—Heading in too many directions keeps you going nowhere!

The third common mistake most people make when setting goals is they're Not Specific. You may have fallen prey to this error in your past. Have you ever thought of owning a home and said to yourself: 'One day, I'm going to be a homeowner.' The more real that vision becomes, the more specific and detailed you find yourself when talking about it. Soon, the statement, I'm going to own a home becomes: "I'm going to own a four bedroom, two bathroom, home that can accommodate overnight guests comfortably and is within walking distance from the beach." Now that's a goal you can see yourself sinking your teeth into! It's no longer vague, someday wish, but a detailed rendering of what you're planning. Goals that are vague and lack luster with no specifics are hard for you to rally behind or become excited about. Also if your heart isn't in it, your mind won't invent it—and you're simply left with a 'goal-less goal,' wondering how your life would be if you were to ever really complete your goals.

The mantra to remember the 'Not Specific' rule is: Specific Thoughts Yield Quicker Results!

Have you ever tried to put together a complex piece of equipment in your home without having the written instructions or guidebook to show you what to do next? Has someone ever handed you a slip of paper advising it has directions on it for you, but you see the directions are non-existent and incoherent?

A great technique to add to this 'Too Many' error is to focus on 'like goals' to complete tasks in one goal set that overlaps into the other. For example; if your goal is to eat healthily and to lose weight, these would can be achieved in the same quarter.

As you begin to consciously choose your foods and incorporate a regimen of 'moving your body more,' and since your goals now go hand in hand, you're able to give your attention to these two goals without feeling it's too much of a stretch. 'Grouping like goals' together allows you to focus your attention properly on moving forward in two separate areas while achieving them both at the same time!

The mantra to remember the 'Too Many' rule is: Too many goals leads to feelings of despair—Heading in too many directions keeps you going nowhere!

The third common mistake most people make when setting goals is they're Not Specific. You may have fallen prey to this error in your past. Have you ever thought of owning a home and said to yourself: 'One day, I'm going to be a homeowner.' The more real that vision becomes, the more specific and detailed you find yourself when talking about it. Soon, the statement, I'm going to own a home becomes: "I'm going to own a four bedroom, two bathroom, home that can accommodate overnight guests comfortably and is within walking distance from the beach." Now that's a goal you can see yourself sinking your teeth into! It's no longer vague, someday wish, but a detailed rendering of what you're planning. Goals that are vague and lack luster with no specifics are hard for you to rally behind or become excited about. Also if your heart isn't in it, your mind won't invent it—and you're simply left with a 'goal-less goal,' wondering how your life would be if you were to ever really complete your goals.

The mantra to remember the 'Not Specific' rule is: Specific Thoughts Yield Quicker Results!

Have you ever tried to put together a complex piece of equipment in your home without having the written instructions or guidebook to show you what to do next? Has someone ever handed you a slip of paper advising it has directions on it for you, but you see the directions are non-existent and incoherent?

The mantra to remember the Not Written error is: Create Goals That Are Truly Exciting—And To Achieve Them, Put Them In Writing!

Now that you know 'The Top-4 Common Mistakes Most People Make When Setting Goals,' ensure that you avoid these pitfalls and have fun using these simple, easy-to-implement practices in your goal-setting regimen. Soon, you'll be able to join the ranks of the percentage of the population that are achieving their goals!

Danielle LaRock

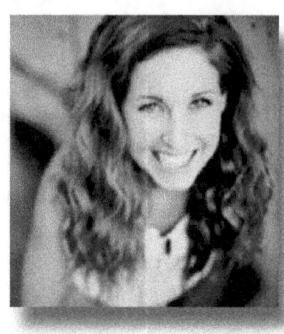

Danielle is Founder of The Haven, an Intuitive Business Coach, and a Spiritual Teacher.

Her vision is creating a world where we see each other for who we truly are and live from our Authentic Selves.

She believes that the world wants the Real You, and when we Discover the Haven Within™ ourselves, we are truly able to live our life of purpose and make our positive impact in this world.

Danielle works with visionary change leaders – individuals who want to make a BIG difference in the world, answer their true calling, and earn and serve abundantly through their healing work.

"Without health, life is not life; it is only a state
of languor and suffering."
~ Francois Rabelais ~

Shepherdstown, West Virginia, USA

Website: www.YourHavenWithin.com

Social Media:
• www.facebook.com/YourHavenWithin

It's time to Answer Your Calling - Your Intuitive Coaching Call at YourHavenWithin.com/Your-Vision

Healing Healers

"**I** don't know what's wrong with me." These were words I kept repeating to myself as my body continued to be unresponsive to any medical treatment – prescription, natural, or otherwise.

I had been battling severe digestive symptoms for four years. They came on suddenly – almost like someone flipped a switch. One day healthy, and bam! The next day, I was in the bathroom 4-10 times a day. With no end in sight.

I was determined to heal, but after countless doctor's visits, a mountain of nutritional and herbal supplements, and a 30-day juice fast, I was running out of ideas.

And hope.

And toilet paper.

I wondered if this was just how I had to live the rest of my life. At age eleven, I was diagnosed with Crohn's disease, an autoimmune disease of the gastrointestinal tract. And I was told there was no cure.

But some part of me believed that there was.

I traveled the world, practiced yoga, meditated, got rubbed down in ayurvedic oil massages, attended months of trainings, and consumed every healing book I could get my hands on.

But it wasn't until I started coaching, that things transformed. ***Radically.***

One of my first ever clients was Mary[1].

1   *Note: All clients' names have been changed to preserve client confidentiality.*

I distinctly remember the day I first coached Mary. There's always a level of awe as I observe this person opening up to me with their greatest fears and dreams.

Mary didn't just want a change. ***She wanted a life transformation.*** She wanted to depart the job at the pharmacy she was working at and embark on something new... something that would allow her that same feeling she felt when she was outside, breathing in the fresh air, feeling that clarity of mind that nature so amply provides. We talked about the possibilities for her new business, how it would affect her relationships, and what this transformation would mean for her.

The last thing she shared with me as we completed our session was, "Yes, maybe this change will help with my colitis."

My jaw dropped.

***

Ray had just been diagnosed with lupus when he came to work with me. He was gearing up to start his own coaching practice, and he had more energy than any man I knew. He would wake up at 4am, get on the treadmill, get his kids off to school, then work 12 hour days at his business for the car dealership. He and his wife would then prepare a vegan meal for their family, and he'd roll into bed, sometimes not until midnight, only to do it all over again.

So he was especially frustrated and at a loss when his body would go into full lockdown and it hurt to even move his fingers. His doctors loaded him up on corticosteroids, causing him to gain weight from the medication, and he then bravely dealt with his own shifting perception of his appearance on top of everything else.

But Ray was determined.

***

I was leading a retreat in Vermont. I crawled into bed one night on day two of the week – a big breakthrough day for everyone – and cracked open Steering by Starlight by Martha Beck, one of the pioneers in the life-coaching field.

It was about halfway through the book that Martha started talking about Madison. Madison was a high-powered Wall Street professional who suddenly started to experience complete exhaustion. Every muscle in her body went into "power down" mode. To the point where even carrying a stack of towels to the bathroom caused pain so extreme, she could hardly move her arms for days.

She kept getting conflicting diagnoses, and no real improvement with treatment.

According to Beck, Madison drew her aside at one of her seminars and said:

> " '…I figured you'd think I was crazy. But I didn't start getting my health back until I started admitting to myself that…' Her voice trailed off…
>
> 'That what?' [Martha] said.
>
> ' That my whole life, I've always know I'm supposed to be some kind of… healer,' said Madison. 'Not medically, more, uh, intuitive.'
>
> She covered her face with her hands. 'I've been fighting this for years,' she whispered. 'I did not go to Yale to become a fruit loop.'" [2]

That night, I had trouble falling asleep.

Martha had introduced me to a puzzle piece that made the picture click.

It's called: Shaman Sickness.

***

"Shaman sickness" actually refers to a well-documented phenomenon. According to anthropologists, in many traditional societies, shamans (also known as druids, medicine people, healers, and empaths) discover their calling after being struck by prolonged, incomprehensible illness, which heals only after they accept the spiritual nature of their vocation and allow themselves to "shamanize."

If I had read this a few years ago, I would have scoffed, rolled my eyes, and thought, "Woo-woo magic," while twirling my finger next to my temple.
But when you experience something, and then begin to see it elsewhere, and then research comes up to smack you in the face, it's a little hard to ignore anymore.
Shaman sickness is an illness, disease, or set of symptoms –mental or physical - that does not respond to normal treatment. The illness is cured only when the healer accepts their gift and steps into their role as a mystic. As a result of this, the individual can work with others who are struggling to cross this same territory.

The healer heals.

Beck, Martha. Steering by Starlight: Find Your Right Life No Matter What. Published by Martha Beck. 2008.

Shamans, contrarians, medicine men/women from all cultures share certain similar characteristics. Typically during childhood, they may be sickly or accident-prone. They are extremely empathetic, sensitive to the emotions of others, and may suffer from high anxiety and/or emotional overload. They may deal with depression or substance abuse issues as a result of being so "wide open." Some have sleeping or waking dreams or visions, and this leads to a life-long interest with the spiritual realm. People tend to be drawn to these visionaries for advice. The challenge is that these healers struggle with anyone understanding them.

How do you know if you are one of these people? See if you resonate with these statements:

> You've always felt a bit…different than everyone else. Odd or outcast even. And yet…you have the ability to help others feel like they are accepted and understood.

> You have this incredible urge that you have something very important to do in this lifetime.

> You have a vision for the world that most cannot see in the current reality.

> Surface level conversations do not interest you. You crave deep connection.

> You've experienced what is sometimes referred to as "the dark night of the soul" – losing a family member, suffering from illness, and/or deep emotional or spiritual turmoil.

You may be reading this and thinking, "Well, I'm sure everyone feels or has experienced this in some way."

Exactly.

Because we are all, in our own unique way, shamans. We are all healers.

The thing is, in western society, with our veneration of modern science, stepping into a role of a mystic can classify you as borderline insane. A true "fruit loop."

So what do we do with the gift? We repress it.

What happens to all that energy? It goes into our body. And gets **stuck**.

Many healers have taught about their personal journey through self-healing, and the resulting work they do with clients. Some notable ones include Louise Hay (teacher and author of *You Can Heal Your Life*, which has sold over 50 million copies world-wide), Amy B Scher (energy therapist and author of the book *This is How I Save My Life*, chronicling her journey of stem cell and energy healing), Bruce Lipton (Scientist and author of *Biology of Belief*, with scientific evidence that energy and environment are what determine our genetic expression), and Carolyn Myss (medical intuitive and author of the acclaimed *Anatomy of the Spirit*), to name just a few.

What do all of the journeys they share have in common?

That not accepting this knowledge, this knowing that we have a *Calling*, drains and weakens us. We start to experience feelings ranging from low-level malaise to addiction, chronic exhaustion, or full-blown body breakdown.

That is, until we decide to claim our true destiny.

***

Mary's and Ray's stories are just an extreme version of breakdowns that I have observed in many of my clients who tell me that in some way, they have lost their purpose.

When you lose sight of why you are here and the unique way you serve the world, it only makes sense that this depletes or weakens your life force.

So what do you do?

Well, you've got to choose, of course.

When I do breakthrough sessions with my clients, there always comes a point where the individual must choose - To heal or not to heal. Do I continue to believe that I am the past self that I have always been? Or do I instead choose to let go of who I thought I once was, in order to become who I might be?

What nudges this choice in the direction of the latter?

A vision that is BIGGER than yourself.

When you have a mission for the world that is bigger than you, bigger even than any one individual you support, you can't help but be in your purpose-lane. And in purpose-lanes, there is no room for sickness. There is no room for misalignment. There is only a deep and true inner knowing, that you are Called to service. And you know it, deep inside of you.

You will do anything to save the world.

Including boldly accepting yourself in the unknown world of the healer.

So what happens to that old story of sickness?

It goes back into the nothingness from whence it came.

***

For the past several months, Ray has been dedicating more of his energy to his passion business, taking down time for himself, and accepting his role as a coach to help others through this process.

Before our breakthrough work together, Ray was blowing up on corticosteroids to manage his illness. A few months ago, Ray dropped down from 20 mg of prednisone to 5 mg.

No symptoms.

In a recent email to me about his miraculous turn around, he wrote:

"Basically, I've chosen health."

***

Mary took a bold step out of her "safe" job and has experienced dramatic reduction in her symptoms, with no use of pharmaceutical drugs. She hikes daily now and reports that she finally feels like she is able to "breathe again." Her renewed sense of freedom has led to increased energy for her new business, helping others with natural remedies and meditation practices to provide healing benefits.

She's an example of how when we continue to align with our authenticity, to take the leap into what we truly desire, that we can't help but want to give. It really demonstrates the age-old adage:

"You live it, to give it."

***

I sat on the hard plastic chair in the super air-conditioned doctor's office. I had taken the day off from coaching to drive an hour to find out the results of my latest test. The door opened and the gastroenterologist strode in, his dictation assistant in tow. As he sat down, I mentally prepared myself for the worst.

"Who diagnosed you?" he asked.

"Well, several doctors since I was eleven. But this is the first colonoscopy I've had in six years," I answered.

He scrolled through the notes on his computer. He looked up, paused, and said frankly:

"You have no signs of Crohn's disease."

Wait, what?

He furrowed his brow. "And you haven't been on any medication for this in the past five years?" he inquired…again. This was the third time he asked me.

"No, none…" I trailed off, as what he was saying totally sank into my mind.
I shuffled out of the doctor's office ten minutes later, clutching the report from the colonoscopy procedure. Two weeks later, I opened my mail from my second opinion, and read "Your blood and stool tests have come back completely normal."

Except I knew. This what anything but normal.

This was healing.

Diane Garrison, Ph.D.

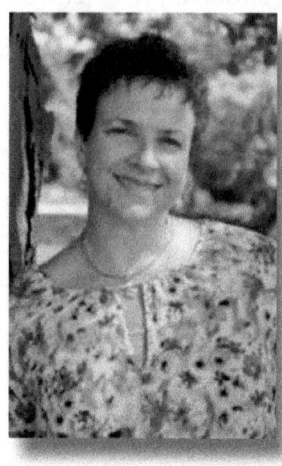

Diane Garrison, Ph.D. is a devoted wife, loving mother, and budding author.

She is a clinical psychologist of 25 years experience. She has worked with clients in individual, group, and workshop settings focusing on many types of challenges including life adjustment, mental health, addiction, spiritual growth, and self-actualization.

In 2013 she opened *Lake Country Wellness & Counseling*, a Holistic Healing Center dedicated to helping each client obtain radiant health and well-being: Mind-Body-Spirit-Emotion.

Through her own personal growth and spiritual transformation, she has come to understand that this work is both her life purpose and mission. She is both honored and grateful to be able to assist others in their healing journey.

"Lack of forgiveness causes almost all
of our self-sabotaging behavior."
~ Mark Victor Hansen ~

Pewaukee, Wisconsin, USA

I am passionate about empowering you to create profound change and personal evolution!

www.LakeCountryWellnessandCounseling.com/

The Power and Grace of Self-Compassion

Self-compassion is a term many of us have heard, but few of us truly understand and practice. It is not taught to us by our culture or even encouraged. Yet it is a very powerful tool and not difficult to learn. I have been a practicing therapist for 25 years and doing my own personal healing work for even longer. I have worked hard to develop a positive relationship with myself. However, it was not until I began studying and practicing "Self-Compassion" these past two years that my deep healing and transformation truly began.

I am a recovering perfectionist and 'achieve-aholic.' My success came from hard work and lots of it. I was constantly driven and not able to truly appreciate or savor my accomplishments. Although I have been receiving spiritual mentoring and practicing meditation for many years, I was still quite self-critical with unrealistic expectations for myself (and others). I was relying on my "masculine strengths" to achieve. I was very controlled, structured, driven, and mentally focused. Self-compassion has helped me tap into my "feminine powers". I am able to be more nurturing, creative, receptive, and heart-centered. It took my body going into serious trauma to wake up and truly see the damage of my Type-A personality style.

I have learned to listen to my body and my heart: what powerful teachers they can be. I listen to my energy. I sense into to my pain, physical and emotional. I notice tension and I notice ease and flow. I am more in tune with my inner voice, my intuition, and I pay attention to the messages of my gut. I now know that I can be kind and gentle to myself and still stand for excellence and self-growth. In fact, it is easier now that I am compassionate towards myself.

So I ask you, why is it so easy to be compassionate to others, yet so hard to be kind to our self? Old programming really. Our cultural training, our Christian tradition, teaches us that it is good to think of others and selfish to think of ourselves. We believe that self-compassion is weak, that it is self-indulgence, or even self-pity. We fear we are letting ourselves off the hook when what we really need is harsh criticism and self-judgment to motivate ourselves to change and just pick ourselves up by our boot straps and carry on. Please recall that **Jesus** tells us to "**Love our neighbor as our self**". This assumes we love our self. Yet we rarely do.

Self-compassion is an emotional response to our own suffering. It is a gentle and understanding reaction to our mishaps, mistakes, and painful life experiences. It is soft and calming. Self-compassion is about embracing our life experiences, whether positive or painful. I believe everything happens for a reason, so let me learn from even the tough incidents.

Self-compassion is a recognition of our common humanity: our imperfections, the things that go wrong in our life, are all part of our shared human experience. Life has pain and everyone experiences it. We are not uniquely flawed or the only one experiencing deep suffering. Anything we have experienced, someone has experienced before. We are not alone.

Self-compassion is also an act of mindfulness, a turning toward our painful emotions and a willingness to sit with them. It is not stuffing our feelings or trying to intellectualize them away by going straight to problem-solving mode. It is not over dramatizing our feelings, nor becoming overwhelmed by them. It is a deliberate, conscious choice to observe with interest and curiosity how our emotions activate sensations in our body (a tightness in the chest, a boiling in the belly) and what information they give to us. Self-compassion is heart centered and tender. It is powerful and very personal. I like to visualize the self-compassion process as the **Loving Parent** in me nurturing the **Vulnerable Child** within.

To get a quick sense of what I am talking about, do this exercise. Sit comfortably in a chair. Close your eyes and slow down your breath, sensing into your body, in space, at this moment. Then gently place your hands, crossed over one another, on your chest, over your heart. Notice the feelings and sensations that this creates... This is a heart hug, a simple act of self-compassion.

The research is very consistent (check out the website of the work of Dr. Kristin Neff, or read her 2011 book "**Self-Compassion**" for more detailed information). Self-compassion increases emotional resilience and decreases anxiety, depression, stress, and perfectionism. It makes one less afraid of failure and more willing to take risks. Self-compassion is related to happiness, optimism, life satisfaction, and self-confidence. People who practice self-compassion are more willing to take responsibility for their mistakes and more willing to apologize for them. People who practice self-compassion are more likely to exercise, stick to diets, quit smoking, and cope well with chronic pain. **Are you convinced yet?**

Here are three ways you can begin the practice of and commitment to self-compassion:

I. Basic Self-Compassion Exercise *[adapted from Neff (2011)]*

This method uses the 3 components of self-compassion: Mindfulness, Awareness of Our Common Humanity, Kindness to Self.

When feeling stress or emotional pain: Close your eyes. Think of the upsetting situation. Rather than going into the storyline, notice what you are feeling, notice were your body is activating, holding the emotion. Mindfully focus on that area of the body and notice the qualities of the energy (e.g. is there a size, or shape, color or weight, movement or texture). You can try to label the emotion (anxiety, anger, etc.), but it is not necessary. Take a few deep breaths. Put your hands over your heart and repeat these phrases until you feel calm. End your practice with three deep cleansing breaths before you open your eyes.

> *This is a moment of suffering*
> *Suffering is a part of life*
> *May I be kind to myself*
> *May I give myself the compassion I need*

Feel free to make the wording more personal: "This hurts", "Pain is a part of life", "May I accept myself as I am", "May I forgive myself", "May I learn to accept what I cannot change".

II. Daily Practices:

These next two exercises can be used daily to cultivate feelings of compassion and loving kindness for yourself. They can also be used like the above exercise in times of stress or self-judgment. Find a quiet place to sit. Close your eyes, take a few deep breaths to center yourself, place your hands over your heart and repeat these phrases until you feel calm. End your practice with three deep cleansing breaths before you open your eyes.

Try practicing one of these exercises for five minutes daily. Try it in the morning to start you day or practice it as you lie in bed waiting to fall asleep.

Loving Kindness Practice *[from Neff (2011), pgs. 203-205]*
- May I feel safe
- May I feel peaceful
- May I be kind to myself
- May I accept myself as I am (or my life as it is)

Hoʻoponopono *(Hawaiian spiritual technique, www.wanttoknow.info)*
- I love you
- I'm sorry
- Please forgive me
- I thank you

Like any new skill, mastering self-compassion will require lots of consistent practice and patience. If you are used to negative self-talk and self-criticism, it will take time to reverse this old pattern. In fact, you may even experience back draft in the beginning, a more fierce presence of negative self-talk. This is normal. This is ego trying to maintain control of your behavior. Simply except it as part of the learning process and give compassion to the ego for its fear of letting go. Let your Higher Self guide your Ego (which is based more on old mental habits and fearful core beliefs than the truth in any situation). Your ego wants to protect the status quo, while your higher self wants you to expand into your personal greatness. Go for the greatness!

As you delve into a steady practice of self-compassion you may discover that your heart center is expanding, that you can be more tender with yourself and others. You may find yourself more aware of your negative thinking patterns and begin seeking ways to challenge these negative beliefs. It is quite possible that you will become more skilled at affirming yourself, choosing positive, deliberate self-talk vs. the negative self-talk that runs on auto-pilot. Turning inward can begin to feel natural and healthy, rather than scary and foreign. You may discover, deep within you, a yearning and passion to develop a loving, honoring relationship with yourself and truly believe it is possible. I know because I am experiencing this and if I can, you can too! (By the way, I teach this to all my clients and it really works for them as well.)

Although self-compassion is a self-care skill and a personal practice, don't be afraid to ask for support in your learning journey. Tell others what you are up to and even share what you are learning. Teach them the self-compassion practices to help you integrate your own skills. If you get stuck, if that negative self-talk is creating pain and overwhelm, don't be afraid to seek professional guidance. We all deserve a helping hand and your health and well-being deserve your time and attention.

I thank you for your kind attention to this topic. I leave you with this this grace filled message. Peace to you always.

Forget About Enlightenment

By: John Welwood

Sit down wherever you are,
And listen to the wind singing in your veins.
Feel the love, the longing, the fear in your bones.
Open your heart to who you are, right now,
Not who you would like to be,
Not the saint you are striving to become,
But the being right here before you, inside you, around you.
All of you is holy.
You are already more and less
Than whatever you can know.
Breath out,
Touch in,
Let go.

References

Neff, K.D. (2011). *Self-compassion. New York: William Morrow.*

Neff, K. D., & Dahm, K. A. (2014). *Self-Compassion: What it is, what it does, and how it relates to mindfulness (pp. 121-140). In M. Robinson, B. Meier & B. Ostafin (Eds.) Mindfulness and Self-Regulation. New York: Springer. PDF http://self-compassion.org/*

Richard Perry

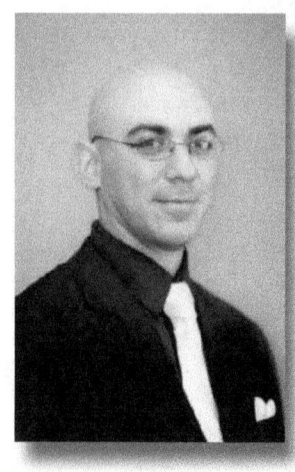

Rich Perry is a coach, corporate trainer, author, and entrepreneur. He was invited by Jim Britt and Jim Lutes to be a co-author in *The Change,* the fastest growing personal development book series in the world, and currently serves as co-host for *The Change Book Radio Show.*

His gift is in his ability to relate to each person and take the client on a hero's journey by integrating both conscious and unconscious performance to create a lasting and powerful change.

Rich works with entrepreneurs and leaders who want to make a difference in the world.

"Everybody can be great . . . because anybody can serve.
You don't have to have a college degree to serve.
You don't have to make your subject and verb agree to serve.
You only need a heart full of grace. A soul generated by love."
~ Rev. Dr. Martin Luther King, Jr. ~

Wilkes-Barre, Pennsylvania, USA

Website: www.thepathofme.com

Social Media:
• www.facebook.com/thepathofme

Get Your FREE eBook – *Finding Purpose in the Unhappiest Place in America + BONUS Mindset Training* - https://www.thepathofme.com

The Silent Torchbearer

What do you envision when you think of a torchbearer? Most likely you picture a person holding a long flaming stick. Perhaps you even elaborated the vision by placing the person deep within a black cave, about to traverse unfamiliar or treacherous terrain at night, or journeying among a group of mystics to a sacred site in order to perform an ancient ceremony. In any case, the torchbearer is the person whose duty it is to light the way for others because without this source of illumination the group would be left to fumble and struggle through the darkness.

It is my belief that we all have a divine inner glow waiting to radiate brilliance out into the world and by no means do I pretend to be alone in believing this to be true as it's commonly shared by countless peoples from various traditions around the globe. As you're reading this book right now, more than likely, you too share this idea. Maybe the reason you chose this book is because you've been feeling a burning sensation in your chest, eager to fuel the fire and figure out how you too can light the way for others as a holistic practitioner, coach, or speaker.

Find Your Inner Glow

The vast majority of people around the globe truly do want to live a meaningful and fulfilling life and contribute something of value to those closest and society as a whole. It's in our nature to connect with others and want to be of service. The main differentiator is whether the person is willing to look within and find their inner glow so that they can begin to light the way for others.

If you're just setting out on this journey then I would encourage you to begin with honesty. What is it about you that lights the room and how can you contribute to the lives of those around you? We all have wonderful qualities about us, however, far too many people keep their abilities hidden and locked away for fear of scorn or criticism. Still others refuse to do anything simply because they doubt their abilities and don't believe that they are enough to make a difference.

"If you think you are too small to make a difference, try sleeping with a mosquito"
~ H.H. the 14th Dalai Lama ~

Finding your true inner glow means uncovering a magnificent gift that you can freely give at any time, over and over again, without depletion. You need only find your personal glow. If you don't know what yours is or the answer is still hazy then simply stand in front of the mirror and ask yourself sincerely and openly. There's going to be one answer that stands out above the rest but if you're back and forth between a few choices then write them down on a piece of paper and repeat each one out loud paying careful attention to how it feels when you say the words. Eventually you'll notice that certain choices create a powerful feeling while others are much weaker so cross those off the list, whittling it down until you have the one that rings true for you.

Holding the Torch

Once you've discovered your gift it's decision time. You must choose whether or not you want to commit to this new course. The choice is yours and yours alone but you must be willing and ready to make the full commitment or stay where you are in life.

During my youth I was very active with the Boy Scouts of America and within the organization is an honored brotherhood known as the Order of the Arrow, which is basically the National Honor Society for Scouts. The Order of the Arrow recognizes those Scouts who demonstrate the ideals of Scouting to the highest degree and utilizes Native American traditions and ceremonies within the society to further encourage chief ideals.

To keep with the nature of the program the initiation and recognition ceremonies are held during special camping trips privately at night and fires and torches are used to add to the mystique. Some camps even have sites used exclusively for these ceremonies so that newcomers are brought into unfamiliar regions, of an otherwise familiar camp, having only the light of the torchbearer to guide the way.

New initiates usually play the part of the torchbearer because it's a non-speaking role of the ceremony however that doesn't mean it's any less significant. In fact, the role has tremendous symbolism and responsibility as it places a Scout in the position to guide a group of his peers through the woods in the darkened night holding a flaming torch. (Don't fret moms and worrywarts because proper fire safety is practiced.)

Similarly, as you journey this bright new path you're sure to find responsibility and privilege in sharing powerful insights and tools with those who are just beginning.

The idea of each *one teach one* holds that we should all do our best to educate, empower, share, and serve others who could benefit especially those who may be less experienced.

This idea was also instilled in me during martial arts studies. Classes were instructed by the *sensei* (teacher) but students were encouraged to seek additional guidance and mentoring from those directly above them in rank. This practice is mutually beneficial because the lesser rank student receives extra support in learning and the ranking student gains the benefit of reinforced learning through teaching the technique, which creates a win/win situation.

It might be in your best interest to adopt this practice and share with others as you acquire new skills and insights because it will help you to relearn the information and strengthen your understanding and grasp of the material. We learn by teaching.

Commitment to Your Cause

This is most important because it will differentiate those that are truly serious from those who are just hobbyists or seminar junkies. If this is your path then you must walk it with full conviction. Being a torchbearer means that you are absolutely committed to the duty. This isn't simply a task to be performed when it's convenient. Either you're willing to unconditionally give yourself to the role or you're just interested in trying something attractive.

We all know those people, the ones that flock to seminars and workshops ready to shell out money and get a brand new fix or stimulation but never willing to dive deep into the rabbit hole and journey within. These individuals love samples, free trials, and test drives but that's as far as they'll ever go, which is okay for them. That's why all-you-can-eat-buffets will never go out of business in America because people love to pick and choose and get a little taste of everything without having to fully commit to making a decision.

Think about someone you know that fits this description. Do you really want this person's advice in anything? Sure s/he might be a jack-of-all-trades but, considering the second part of the saying, this person is probably not the ideal candidate to guide the journey that will define your life. That being said, as a torchbearer people will be placing their trust in you and your expertise. Don't they deserve the best service and direction possible?

Being committed means actually doing it verses trying to do it. The world doesn't need any more samplers or triers; it needs more doers. Once you know your passion and you've found your glow then do it. Don't touch your toes to the water or gently wade in because you're afraid to get hit by the waves. Jump right in! Feel this new world around you, experience it, and embrace it. You owe it to yourself and others to be fully dedicated to this way of life.

Commitment also means following through with a particular course of action and doing it to the best of your ability. You don't have to be the best but you do have to do your absolute best. There's a big difference. Don't concern yourself with being perfect or stay in the shadows until you've reached elite status because far too many people fall short of their perfectionist aspirations and then they give up for failing to live up to their unrealistic expectations.

The true and loyal torchbearer takes this pledge knowing that there might come a time when a spark or ember will fall from the flame, landing on skin. This will probably burn you for a moment. You'll experience this in the form of hard work, sacrifice, and having to do the things that you don't necessarily want to do in order to achieve the desired goal. Do you have the tenacity to stand strong devoted to your personal obligation? Hopefully you do. Remember, anything worthwhile requires a sincere and steadfast decision plus matching effort and follow through to the end.

And They'll Say You Changed

Now here is the portion of the story that most people won't acknowledge however I feel it would be a great disservice and deception through omission to leave it out. As you position yourself to guide others through unfamiliar territory journeying towards an unknown destination, you might be questioned or criticized by those in your charge. In fact, if you're doing your job properly then you'll surely experience resistance from peers. It sounds odd to say but it's true.

Most people fear change and would prefer to stay in the safety of their comfort zone. While they might initially show interest or intrigue, eventually they will question or criticize whether you know what you are doing, which is why a deep personal level of commitment is so important because you must remain strong during this period. Let your actions and perseverance be your response. This is another reason, symbolically, why the torchbearers in our Scouting ceremonies were silent roles because the guide's duty was to lead his peers by illumined action to the promised destination.

As you walk this new path, those closest to you might even accuse you of not being the same person anymore and say that you've changed. Well... good, because you have changed! Take it as a compliment and thank them for noticing. This is where the majority of people fall short because they all want the status of being a torchbearer in moments of glory when accolades are being dished out but not when hardships arise. For better or worse, it only makes sense that when times are darkest, people will turn to those with the light for the answer. The triers, seminar junkies, and jack-of-all-trades type individuals are usually the first to shy away from responsibility because they know they aren't willing to make a true comment to a chosen path. It's much easier to walk behind the light hand in pocket than it is to stand tall holding the flame high enough for all to see.

The Lighthouse

In antiquity people would signal ships with raised fires and for hundreds of years these lighthouses served as entrance markers guiding mariners to port. Before clearly defined seaports were established, and long before modern navigation systems, the ships needed a way of not only identifying land but having a way to safely come to harbor and an elevated light source was the answer.
Just as these fires lit up the sky welcoming ships to come in for needed supplies or trade, you too should be a source of light for those you encounter in life. Of course not every passing ship will choose to dock and some might only stay for a brief amount of time but this still holds a wonderful opportunity to connect and exchange with like-minded individuals.

Keep in mind that the lighthouse didn't use flashy signs begging crews to come in nor did the attendant physically bring the ship in doing the captain's job for him. Everyone has his/her job and each job maintains designated responsibilities. You would do well to know your unique duties and commit to doing your absolute best at all times. Now is your time to be the beacon of light for others who are searching.

Light the Way

We can all be torchbearers in our own way. It only takes the decision to do so and the commitment to adhere to the responsibilities of raising the flame. How can you serve others and light the way on the journey ahead?

If you've ever had to light a series of candles then you know that you only need one match because once the first candle is lit you can use its flame to ignite the others. Your words and purpose can be the spark of inspiration for those in your community while your actions guide them in finding a more fulfilling and prosperous life. Be the torchbearer for the next person in line and a leader for those who follow you.

Deborah Crowe

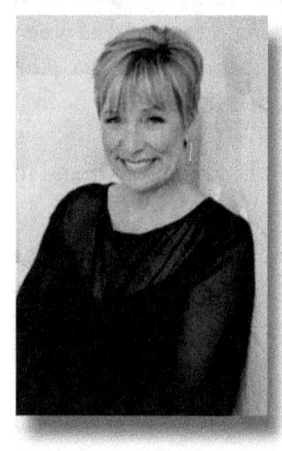

"Work Life Balance is not a trend, it's a lifestyle"
- Deborah Crowe

As the CEO of a successful medical case management practice for 23 years, I recognized the growing need for further supports for professionals and families dealing with catastrophic illnesses and the need for stress management.

Leading with this new vision, I have evolved into a Work Life Balance Specialist and I've created a model for revitalization, stress management, and leadership success.

I provide coaching to women, men, and couples and I absolutely enjoy working with companies (small to large) to assist with their EAP programs and work with their HR department to reduce and eliminate short-term disability claims and get the balance back to employees and be the mediator between the employer and employee.

My ultimate goal is to get ahead of the curve and educate employers about the importance of work-life balance so that employees do not become so stressed, receive a medical diagnosis and go off work on short-term disability.

"You don't have to make yourself miserable to be successful.
It's natural to look back and mythologize the long nights and manic moments
of genius, but success isn't about working hard, it's about working smart."
~ Andrew Wilkinson ~

London, Ontario, Canada

Website: www.debcrowe.com

Social Media:
- www.twitter.com/LetsGetBalanced
- www.facebook.com/deb.crowe/

If this chapter resonates with you, let's chat about helping you integrate and sustain Work-Life Fit

I've Found the Unbalance

I live in a beautiful city called London, located in a breathtakingly beautiful province called Ontario and a country I am so proud to live in Canada.

Each day I awake with a mantra to "be a miracle". This allows me to start my day with gratitude and be the best version of myself and always serving others any way I can.

As a member of my community, I volunteer at St. Joseph's Hospice. This experience on a weekly basis honors my soul as it's a true gift and quite frankly a privilege to be part of someone's life when they reach the stage of palliative care.

Recently, I completed a six week course on grief and bereavement. A small glimpse into the world of Thanatology. During the course we were often asked how many times our friends and family would say things like, "How can you volunteer there, isn't it depressing". Each week I ruminated on this question and it certainly evoked many different emotions for me.

Then...the AHA moment occurred....

This is the true representation in all our lives. This is the '**unbalance**'. Trauma, loss, death, injury.... we are not born with the innate ability to just "deal" with these things. They come unexpected and everyone reacts to them differently.

As a medical case manager for over 23 years, I witnessed how the human spirit reacts to such loss. Some people cry and are inconsolable, others laugh (as a nervous reaction and their inability to know what to do), and some people keep themselves so busy that they describe it as a "numb" stage and the barrier to allow them not to "think" or "feel". My point is we, as human beings react to loss and trauma in many different ways.

The 'unbalance' occurs as sometimes we cannot get ourselves back on track. There is no time lineage. I have seen and heard many times someone say, Well, it›s been two years, surely you're over this by now, or my favorite comment is «I can›t believe they have moved forward, as (person who has passed) has only been gone for a year.

In our course, we were taught some beautiful strategies such as:

1. Not to judge, to just allow

2. Not to speak, to just listen

3. Lean in and show your genuine ability to care

4. There is no time lineage, it's a journey of healing

5. Silence is sometimes the best strategy

6. Crying can be a cleansing for the soul

7. Many emotions are shown, allow what is to be

8. Each support group will vary

9. Allow your loved one the space they need

10. Be present in all capacities (physical, emotional, spiritual, psychological)

So, I ask that the next time you or someone you love experiences a loss or trauma, embrace the 'unbalance' and allow what is to be.

The takeaway this week is that sometimes you have to embrace the 'unbalance' for a period of time that is unknown. The good news is work life balance always returns when the time is right.

Donate or volunteer for your Hospice if this resonates with you on any level. It's life-changing: http://www.sjhospicelondon.com/

Look to your health; and if you have it, praise God, and value it next to a good conscience; for health is the second blessing that we mortals are capable of; a blessing that money cannot buy.
~ Izaak Walton ~

David Fife

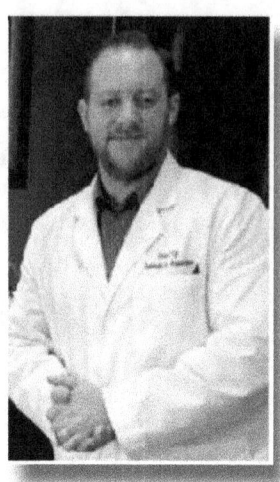

David Fife L.Ac. is a fully-qualified acupuncturist, certified by the National Certification Commission of Acupuncture and Oriental Medicine (NCCAOM) in the United States, licensed in the State of Wisconsin, and practicing at Lake Country Acupuncture.

After graduating with honors from the London College of Traditional Acupuncture in 2005, he went on to study at the Traditional Chinese Medicine Hospital in Hong Zhou, China.

He also had the opportunity to study with renowned masters of ancient Chinese healing and martial arts all across China.

David Fife has personally treated over 10,000 patients in the greater Milwaukee area, and has been a certified acupuncturist for over 10 years.

"Health is the greatest possession.
Contentment is the greatest treasure.
Confidence is the greatest friend.
Non-being is the greatest joy."
~ Laozi ~

Pewaukee, Wisconsin, USA

Website: www.lakecountryacu.com/

Lake Country Acupuncture can help you with your stubborn health concerns. Call for a free treatment!

Acupuncture and Health

When we think of medicine in this country we immediately think of illness. Granted, we cannot have a remedy without a problem but our minds have been carefully conditioned to consider medicine as a means of treating a dis- ease and not one of maintaining and stabilizing health. One cannot be blamed for this. We are constantly bombarded with articles and advertisements about the next revolutionary drug and are encouraged to suggest to our doctors the prescription that they should be giving us.

How many times have you heard, "Ask your doctor about...?" It seems commonplace in our world. If I have this symptom then I'd better take this drug to treat that symptom. Logical right? Point A to point B. Or is it? Maybe, just maybe we are looking at medicine and healthcare in a very rudimentary and linear way. What is truly behind our health and our wellness? What do we need to truly stay well? What is the right medicine? Furthermore, what is the right mindset to have?

Our bodies are quite miraculous. They are constantly healing and replenishing themselves in every way shape and form. The health problems we develop almost always are because of a malfunctioning in a system or systems that otherwise function normally. This "disease process" can happen for a number of different reasons.

Imbalance is something that seems to prevail in this world. There are so many ways we can become imbalanced and subsequently unwell. In Chinese medicine we believe there are both internal and external causes for one's imbalance.

The internal causes are those of the emotional responses to certain stimulus in our environment. What we call internal pernicious influences. They can range from anger and resentment, jealousy, and worry, to being overly excitable or easily startled and chronically fearful. These emotional responses are imbalanced when the system that generates them is imbalanced. If we have a poor lifestyle, are constantly stressed, eat empty or processed food, and constantly surround ourselves with trying situations we will weaken the foundation our body and minds rely upon in order to healthily respond to environmental stimuli. The key to conquering imbalance and disease is to nourish the source. A medical practitioner cannot take stress away but we can certainly guide an individual in the right direction to build up resistance to stress and respond appropriately to it.

There are also external influences. These range from the food we eat and what we drink to the very nature of our surroundings. From our environmental climate to the people we surround ourselves with, as well as, how we organize our household. Again, the stimulus can be adjusted and that is part of the whole equation but we need to strengthen our resistance to these stimuli in order to prevail. In short, we need to have optimal system function in order to deal with life otherwise it will generate illness and survival will be in peril.

Our bodily organs control our bodily function. Health is only possible when all of our organ systems are functioning properly. Other than trauma, illness occurs for two reasons. One is because we are susceptible to illness. If our functional defense is down we are open to invasion. The second reason is functional loss. When a system is not functioning well, then it cannot deal with what is required of it well enough to sustain health. Therefore, it is of the utmost importance that we maintain and sustain bodily function and feed our defense systems to maintain health. So the question is, how do we do this? Simply, we give our bodies what they need.

That comes with the obvious fundamentals for good health. A whole- food-based, well-rounded nutritious diet, avoiding processed and refined foods, drinking plenty of clean water, exercising regularly, and getting ample rest. These are essential. However sometimes these essential pieces are not possible because of underlying malfunction. For example. If you can't shut your mind down at night, how can you sleep properly? If you have significant inflammation and pain in your knee, how can you stay efficiently active? Thankfully there is another functional tool that has been used by billions of people for thousands of years that can address these issues and many other underlying problems. Most people, certainly in the western world, have very little understanding of this system of medicine and its ability to stimulate optimal function in the human body. This tool is called Acupuncture.

Acupuncture is the insertion of hair thin needles into certain points around the body. When this insertion takes place a number of interesting things happen. Immediately the nervous system is signaled. Depending on the placement of the needles we are able to stimulate specific nervous channels. In doing this, we encourage the movement of circulation along with it. So in actuality, we are moving circulation of blood and energy into the area of the body where it is needed. Blood is a major waste removal tool and when stimulated it will break down obstruction of all kinds. Whether it's inflammation, which most times it is, or if it is tension in the nerve or some form of fluid congestion, moving circulation through these areas will remove obstruction and restore smooth function. More than this, when circulation is encouraged into an area via the acupuncture stimulus, oxygen, nutrients, and hormones will get into the system where they are needed in order to strengthen the function of that given system.

The majority of disease is because of congestion and stagnation within a certain system or because the area in question is weak and functioning poorly as a result. By stimulating circulation we can resolve the overall majority of health problems, because that is what is needed to heal. Without it we cease to be.

The human body is amazingly versatile but even so it can become weakened by years of abuse. If we eat refined sugars and oils for many years we will generate weaknesses in our digestive systems. If we endure intense stress day in day out it will affect our adrenal system, liver and cardiovascular system. Over time even our bodies succumb to poor choices. The great news is our bodies will heal 100 times quicker than they will become ill. If we stimulate otherwise complacent nerves in parts of our body that are weakened or congested we can get the essential healing elements via the circulation into these problematic areas, whatever they may be, and the body's function goes up and our bodies heal!

The time it takes for a person to heal with the use of acupuncture varies from individual to individual, but once it has, we continue to use it to maintain the integrity of our health. For thousands of years in China the Acupuncture physicians were paid if the patient in question was well, not if they were sick! This seems like the reverse of our current conventional model, wouldn't you say?! In our practice we will get a person well and then maintain their wellness. Frequency of treatment becomes far less necessary once the body is doing the work.

Acupuncture is a tool and a very effective one at that. Acupuncture has been body. When this insertion takes place a number of interesting things happen. Immediately the nervous system is signaled. Depending on the placement of the needles we are able to stimulate specific nervous channels. In doing this, we encourage the movement of circulation along with it. So in actuality, we are moving circulation of blood and energy into the area of the body where it is needed. Blood is a major waste removal tool and when stimulated it will break down obstruction of all kinds. Whether it's inflammation, which most times it is, or if it is tension in the nerve or some form of fluid congestion, moving circulation through these areas will remove obstruction and restore smooth function. More than this, when circulation is encouraged into an area via the acupuncture stimulus, oxygen, nutrients, and hormones will get into the system where they are needed in order to strengthen the function of that given system.

The majority of disease is because of congestion and stagnation within a certain system or because the area in question is weak and functioning poorly as a result. By stimulating circulation we can resolve the overall majority of health problems, because that is what is needed to heal. Without it we cease to be.

The human body is amazingly versatile but even so it can become weakened by years of abuse. If we eat refined sugars and oils for many years we will generate weaknesses in our digestive systems. If we endure intense stress day in day out it will affect our adrenal system, liver and cardiovascular system. Over time even our bodies succumb to poor choices. The great news is our bodies will heal 100 times quicker than they will become ill. If we stimulate otherwise complacent nerves in parts of our body that are weakened or congested we can get the essential healing elements via the circulation into these problematic areas, whatever they may be, and the body's function goes up and our bodies heal!

The time it takes for a person to heal with the use of acupuncture varies from individual to individual, but once it has, we continue to use it to maintain the integrity of our health. For thousands of years in China the Acupuncture physicians were paid if the patient in question was well, not if they were sick! This seems like the reverse of our current conventional model, wouldn't you say?! In our practice we will get a person well and then maintain their wellness. Frequency of treatment becomes far less necessary once the body is doing the work.

Acupuncture is a tool and a very effective one at that. Acupuncture has been improves and the acupuncture brings them substantial relief and correction of their health concerns. It happens over and over again.

Pure and simple the body heals itself and acupuncture encourages and increases this possibility immensely. All we need to do is keep exploring our world and see what lies beyond our own self-imposed limitations. The World Health Organization recognizes acupuncture's effectiveness in the treatment of over fifty different medical conditions, and as more research comes out, that list continues to grow.

I have been to China on two separate occasions and witnessed the medicine first hand. I was fortunate enough to work as an intern at the Hong Zhou Traditional Chinese Medicine Hospital in Hong Zhou China and was able to witness the miraculous things that they do to help patients deal with paralysis as a result of a stroke. There were patients that had suffered complete paralysis of one side of their body. Acupuncture was administered 6-7 days a week. In several case,s within a matter of 5-6 months, the paralysis was gone!

Frequency is the key to get the body to heal when it comes to anything. In these cases, the frequent stimulation of the needles in specific areas of the body brought enough blood and energy circulation back to the paralyzed nerves that they started functioning efficiently again. Again, our bodies do a lot more than we give them credit for day to day.

We are seeing acupuncture become more and more accepted in the west. I encourage anyone that is open to living their lives with more vitality and stronger functionality to try acupuncture. All it takes is that first step in a self-explorative direction. You will be pleasantly surprised.

I am amazed at how many people, who discredit acupuncture, have had little to no experience with it at all! This is a common trait. The less we know of something the more we avoid or fear its presence. It is a very rudimentary base level reaction in the human brain. Really, the only cure for this is jumping in head first and experiencing acupuncture, or anything that you lack the experience in that could otherwise enrich your life for that matter. You will certainly be amazed at what you might find out! It may even change your life for the better.

Once we use acupuncture to stimulate our own body's innate ability to heal, our mindset changes. We truly realize how amazing our systems are and that maintenance is the key to long, healthy and happy lives. Once you see it for yourself you will know the amazing power your body has to heal and you will continue to change the minds of others. Pills and surgery are not the only answers, we have other options.

Dr. Matt Frahm

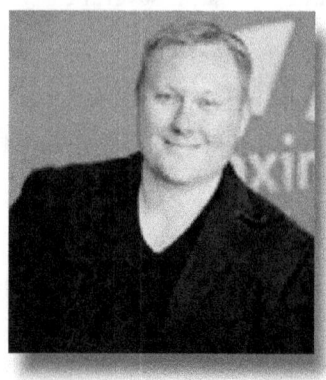

Dr. Matt Frahm is the owner and head doctor at Max Health Chiropractic. Max Health Chiropractic was founded in 2008 in Brookfield, WI to help people avoid unnecessary sickness and disease.

Because of the results thousands of patients have seen, Max Health Chiropractic has grown to 3 locations in the greater Milwaukee area, and Dr. Frahm has been featured on Fox 6, TBN, WTMJ & WISN as Milwaukee's health expert on topics ranging from weight loss, chronic disease prevention, fatigue, hormone imbalance and much more.

Dr. Frahm was also at the 2012 Olympics caring for the US Wrestling Team and has a vision to transform the lives of families across the greater Milwaukee area.

"The patient should be made to understand that he or she must take charge of his own life. Don't take your body to the doctor as if he were a repair shop."
~ Quentin Regestein ~

Brookfield, Wisconsin, USA

Website: www.maxhealthchiro.com

Social Media:
- www.facebook.com/maxhealthchiropractic
- www.twitter.com/mlmke

Remove the interferences that are keeping you from reaching your maximum health potential. www.maxhealthchiro.com

Changing the World Through Healthcare

After traveling to New York City for my daughter Hannah's eighth birthday, I found myself fascinated with the broad spectrum of people, places and events throughout the city. If you've ever visited New York City then you know what I mean; skyscrapers, Broadway shows, luxury hotels, yachts and helicopters mixed-in with street vendors, sidewalk entertainers, homeless people sleeping in the streets and everything in-between. Many times we take life for granted - we assume there will be enough money to pay the bills, food on the table for our next meal and that our health will sustain us to take on the challenges of a new day.

Despite our best efforts to enjoy life to its fullest, there are still areas that we will inevitably take for granted. So how do we decide where to focus our time? What areas of life do we allow to fade? My personal belief is that each person has to come to that conclusion on his or her own. What is that goal? Fulfillment? Or is it success? Or Happiness? Enlightenment? The answer is you're right. At the end of the day if we haven't left this world a better place for the next generation then I personally believe we have failed as a society. After caring for thousands of families, there is one area of life that stands out above the rest. I think we both can agree that the greatest positive change we can make in this world for future generations is by changing the way we view and manage our health as a society.

My goal is to help you achieve all of the above by navigating you through the process of identifying and protecting your greatest asset in creating change in the world, your health. Not your property, not your bank account, not your family, and not your time. Talk about a big, audacious, and feather-ruffling claim! But let me help you understand why I not only believe, but know, this as your greatest asset.

First, health is the area of life that too many people take for granted and therefore end up losing well before they've had the opportunity to make their greatest contribution to the world. Here's a perfect example: my good friend Jim lost his father to a heart attack when he was just a teenager. His father was only 45 years old. Jim's family was obviously devastated and three young boys were left to navigate the world without their father. Tragically, Jim's mother had a stroke a few short years later and now requires live-in nursing assistance to help with her daily routine. Jim and his brothers have had to learn how to provide for their mother's medical expenses plus the monthly household bills associated with raising their own families. Of course they are happy to be in a position financially to help, but the strain on the family relationships, time and resources have taken their toll and caused unnecessary hardships. Jim now recognizes that his family could have avoided much of this unnecessary suffering if they would have developed a better plan for their health.

Jim's family grew up the way many of us did. Meals consisted of refined, processed, sugar-loaded cereals for breakfast, sandwiches for lunch and meat and potatoes for dinner. They thought they were living healthy. They didn't keep junk-food in the house, they were active with the kids in sports, mom and dad made sure everyone got a good night's sleep, they went to church most weekends, and they even served at the local soup kitchen. Jim's family was your prototypical American family. The way they treated their health was no different. Jim remembers going to the pediatrician for yearly physicals and vaccinations. Antibiotics were administered whenever someone in the family fell ill and the family doctor was well liked and trusted in the community. However, no one actually taught them how to protect their health. Like most American families, if you asked Jim where health comes from or how to define health, the answer was quite vague. The most common responses that I hear are as follows:

- I judge my health based on how I feel.
- I know I'm healthy because I "eat right" and "exercise."
- I base my health on how I look.
- Good genes run in my family so I know I'm healthy.
- Bad genes (heart disease, stroke, cancer, etc.) run in my family so I schedule yearly physicals, mammograms, prostate checks, etc. to reduce my risk of the same health issues.

The bottom-line is that Jim's family, and many other American families, take their health for granted. When you take your health for granted, whether knowingly or unknowingly, it will only be a matter of time before you lose your health. The more we take an area of life for granted, the higher the probability we will be negatively impacted by the dysfunction in that area of life. This is certainly true of health more than any other area of life. Once you lose your health, or a close family member loses their health, then, consequently, every other area of life is negatively impacted. This is the second reason why I know health is your greatest asset. When we lose our health, every other area of life is negatively impacted because of how our health plays such an intricate role in every area of living.

The third reason health is your greatest asset is because it reaps the greatest return on investment. I hate to define health in business terms, but it seems to make sense to do so in making my case here. An investment into your health today to maintain it at a high level or to improve it so that you have more energy, more productivity, more motivation, better control of your emotions, better sleep, better sex, and more is the precise reason why its the best investment. Great health is endlessly rewarding which also makes it so easy to take for granted because so many are content to just reap the rewards from the current level of health that they are experiencing. But what if there was more? A level of health that you've never tapped into because you weren't even aware that it existed?

Now that you desire amazing health, we should probably define what health actually means. Is it medications? No. More Medications? No. Vaccinations? No. Surgery? No. So how do you define health? Where does health come from since it certainly doesn't come from any of the previously mentioned sources? The best working definition of health that I have found is from the World Health Organization - physical health is not merely the absence of sickness and disease, but the body's ability to adapt and function at its fullest potential.

In order to be as healthy as possible, we must support the body's ability to adapt and function at its best. Seems obvious, right? But how do we actually do that? What controls adaptation and function within the body? The answer lies in the fact that every single person is empowered with the ability to heal. The power to heal is exactly what keeps us adapting and functioning at our best. It's the same power that brought two cells together inside a mother's womb and, over the course of forty weeks, forms a human being. It's the same power that organizes cells into heart tissue that will pump blood for decades, lung tissue that allows the exchange of oxygen and carbon dioxide, eyes that can see, ears that can hear, and systems that work in harmony, while all functioning without a second thought from our conscious brain.

This is the second reason why I know health is your greatest asset. When we lose our health, every other area of life is negatively impacted because of how our health plays such an intricate role in every area of living.

The third reason health is your greatest asset is because it reaps the greatest return on investment. I hate to define health in business terms, but it seems to make sense to do so in making my case here. An investment into your health today to maintain it at a high level or to improve it so that you have more energy, more productivity, more motivation, better control of your emotions, better sleep, better sex, and more is the precise reason why its the best investment. Great health is endlessly rewarding which also makes it so easy to take for granted because so many are content to just reap the rewards from the current level of health that they are experiencing. But what if there was more? A level of health that you've never tapped into because you weren't even aware that it existed?

Now that you desire amazing health, we should probably define what health actually means. Is it medications? No. More Medications? No. Vaccinations? No. Surgery? No. So how do you define health? Where does health come from since it certainly doesn't come from any of the previously mentioned sources? The best working definition of health that I have found is from the World Health Organization - physical health is not merely the absence of sickness and disease, but the body's ability to adapt and function at its fullest potential.

In order to be as healthy as possible, we must support the body's ability to adapt and function at its best. Seems obvious, right? But how do we actually do that? What controls adaptation and function within the body? The answer lies in the fact that every single person is empowered with the ability to heal. The power to heal is exactly what keeps us adapting and functioning at our best. It's the same power that brought two cells together inside a mother's womb and, over the course of forty weeks, forms a human being. It's the same power that organizes cells into heart tissue that will pump blood for decades, lung tissue that allows the exchange of oxygen and carbon dioxide, eyes that can see, ears that can hear, and systems that work in harmony, while all functioning without a second thought from our conscious brain.

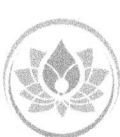

"All the money in the world can't buy you back good health"
~ Reba McEntire ~

Heddy Keith & Keridak Silk

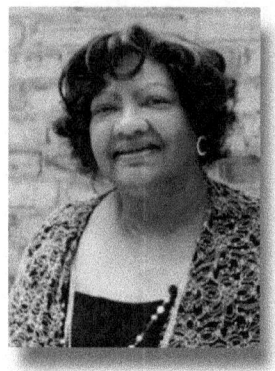

I am a certified hypnotherapist/ Instructor for the National Guild of Hypnotists and the owner of HK Hypnosis, LLC. I earned a Bachelor's degree in Education from the University of Wisconsin-Milwaukee, and a Master's in Education from Cambridge College- Cambridge, MA. I am trained and certified in the Emotional Freedom Technique (EFT) and Hypno-Wav- ing.

She can be reached at Heddykeith51@att.net or call 414-241-2563 for a free phone consultation.

Milwaukee, Wisconsin, USA

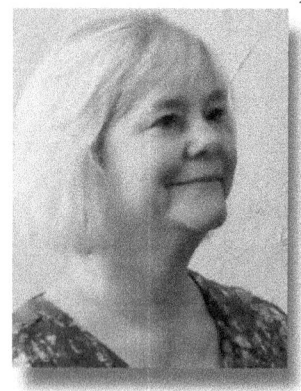

I am an Intuitive Counselor. I am skilled in counseling techniques (Masters from National Louis University), life coaching skills , Reiki Trained. I have fully stepped into my natural abilities as an intuitive.

Contact her at keridakkae@gmail.com 262-404-7119 or 303-887-6477

Menomonee Falls, Wisconsin, USA

"To acquire true self-power you have to feel beneath no one,
be immune to criticism and be fearless."
~ Deepak Chopra ~

Discover Your Power

What can elicit my self-power?

Heddy: Hypnosis helps create a change in mind and attitude and that is the key to changing behavior. It empowers, a person to solve their own problems. The newest clinical research reveals that when used properly, hypnosis and hypnotic suggestion can alter cognitive processes such as memory and pain perception. The aim of hypnosis is self-healing and self-change.

Keridak: You have unlimited potential to change your life. I understand that sometimes this is difficult to understand and difficult to practice. We are all made up of energy. This is proven by physics but has been the basis of religious practices for ages. Energy can be tapped into by our minds. The skills to do this can be taught. Needing help is very common. We are taught by society to deny our body/mind/spirit connection.

Can people really change?

Heddy: It takes courage to change. Yes, people can change when they are ready to deal with their issues. Hypnosis can make a dramatic shift in your life circumstances if you want to change. You are the controlling factor, through your own effort your desired change occurs.

Keridak: Yes. Everything changes; it is up to you what direction that change takes. Understand that this is not who you are. It takes a desire to have a happier, more fulfilled and powerful life. For some just realizing the desire can create the change. Consider the person who lifts an unimaginable weight off of another in a spurt of desire to help. The desire sparks adrenaline and it taps into the Universal Energies. It is amazing what humans can do when they have a desire.

It's been a lifetime of challenges; can I change?

Heddy: Yes, challenges help you grow and reach self-actualization. I look at life as one huge classroom. Maybe it's because I am a teacher, but to me every experience is an opportunity to learn and grow; each challenge you accept and overcome moves you to a higher level like a pyramid game. We learn from tough challenges. Failure leads to success. Walt Disney was told he didn't have imagination, but that didn't stop him.

Keridak: You came into this world with challenges and abilities. Some of those challenges seem insurmountable right now. Some challenges you have conquered only to have that same pattern repeat. Each of us has a unique path we came here to follow. It is important to understand that that path is not set in stone. You have the power to make astounding changes and to free yourself of the challenges of a lifetime. This is the true lesson.

Are thoughts really important?

Heddy: Yes thoughts are the most important thing when speaking of changing behavior. It all begins with your thoughts. You're the director, you create your life with the thoughts you entertain in your mind. The subconscious mind is a powerful tool that we use every day to manage and control our lives. The conscious mind commands and the subconscious mind obeys, it works twenty-four hours a day to make sure your behavior fits the pattern of your thoughts and desires. Thoughts can grow flowers or weeds, they are the seeds you plant and nurture repeatedly in your mind. What you think is what you get.

Keridak: Absolutely! Everything is a reflection of your thoughts. Look at the work by Dr. Masaru Emoto – Messages in Water. He placed words next to a jar of water. Froze it and looked at the crystal structure under a microscope. Words like hate and anger made ugly crystals. The same water with words such as beautiful or love created gorgeous crystals. We are mainly made up of water. Don't worry about the one or two stray thoughts, we all have those. Instead be mindful of the way your typical thoughts flow. Are they focused on anxiety or fears? Do they make you feel hopeful or strong? Is there anger or an underlying feeling of stress? Thoughts can be changed. Changing your thoughts can dramatically change your life.

How can I use the Law of Attraction?

Heddy: What you think about is what you get. The law of attraction says you draw into your life what you repeatedly think about. So why not think about what you want in your life. If you want to be happy, think happy thoughts. If you want a better job sit down and write a description of the kind of job you want? How much money you want to make? How many hours will you work? How much vacation? And what work conditions do you want? Think about the kind of boss you want to work for. In other words make the details specific. According to Buddha, "All that we are is a result of what we have thought." Think about it for a moment, what have you been thinking about?

Keridak: The Law of Attraction is one of several Universal Laws. It means that you control what happens to you by what you think. Have you ever thought something and then had it happen? Sometimes this is a form of Deja Vu or Precognition (spirit messages/dreams telling you what is to come). Other times you have communicated what you want to have happen and it comes to you. The Secret is a popular movie that gives examples of how this can work for people. The more you flex the muscle of receiving what you desire the stronger it becomes.

Are our bodies self-healing?

Heddy: The subconscious mind controls the body. Research as shown that when we speak positive words to plants they grow. George Washington Carver talked to his plants and they grew. I have talked to my dying houseplants and they came back to life. We know the effects negativity have on children, they grow up with low self-worth and lack of self-confidence. "Sticks and stones will break your bones, but names will never hurt you," is a lie. As a person thinks in his subconscious mind, so is he. Being called negative names ends up stored in a child's subconscious mind and he or she grows up believing they are the truth.

Your subconscious mind can heal, empower, inspire, and strengthen you. Everything starts in the mind including disease. Negative thoughts emerge as negative experiences.

Keridak: Absolutely. I have talked about how our thoughts can change what comes to us. Healing is something that you can manifest. Our society teaches the opposite. It makes you feel that you do not have control over your body. There is research that in case after case people have gone beyond what medical science has said was impossible. In many cases, changing mindset, learning to reduce stress, and harnessing universal energy can change your health.

Allan Wich

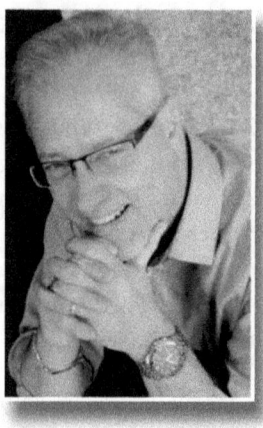

Four open-heart surgeries, one artificial heart valve, one cardiac arrest, dead for 26-minutes, shocked eight times, twelve cardiac injections, and one implanted pacemaker/defibrillator.

Bankrupt, but in the same year made a million dollars.

I triumph over struggle with the courage and gratitude God gave me.

Two traits keep me aligned; my ability to think bold and anticipate.

My large imagination and ability to anticipate growth and change, even disruption helped me realize many goals.

Rarely do I shy from risk if the idea is in direct harmony with my mission, and if it has the ability to provide exponential abundance.

"Cheerfulness is the best promoter of health and is as friendly to the mind as to the body."
~ Joseph Addison ~

Gresham, Oregon, USA

Website: www.allanwich.com

Social Media:
• www.facebook.com/allan.wich

To hear my story, learn more about how to craft and deliver your story, how to create your public artifacts and your homepage, visit me at: www.allanwich.com

How to become Relevant and Visible to a Global Audience

There comes a time in the lives of those who are destined to become great where they must ask themselves, are they living in the shadows of their own capability or are they living their life creating perpetual abundance to the magnitude they were born with, and is that story being told?

RELEVANT

Relevant: having significant and demonstrable bearing upon the matter at hand.

Many are looking for a way to become more personally empowered, personally developed, but often don't know what that looks like, and end up succumbing to the riskless motion of the masses. We have to keep our eyes and hearts open to acknowledging who we are and who we want to become, otherwise we remain stagnant.

What keeps us from a life of abundance is in large part laziness. We find ourselves detached and desensitized. Our ignorance to learning about change can leave us empty and full of regret. We aspire for greatness but live in the minutia of repetition and indifference. Instead of experiencing the vastness of our potential we become selfish, and like a cancer, selfishness is conditioned to engorge itself on its environment leaving little space for healing, growth and abundance. To seek a life of great influence and contribution, one must risk ridicule and rejection by deciding to be heard, often in the face of resistance and conformity.

We are not intended to be aimless in our works and numb to responsibility and opportunity; rather we should stand apart and meet our lives with presence of mind, purpose, power and gratitude. If we do this we will experience an inner glow, peace and accomplishment that will guide us. We must spend our life with the realization that we are to be in the moment, experience life at each and every turn without ignoring our responsibility to contribute; otherwise we risk descent into the listless wandering life of slavery and mediocrity. We must awaken ourselves from the monotony of a daily existence. We are tooled from greatness for greatness, but somewhere along the way we surrendered that right, succumbed to the road most traveled and often find ourselves the absent student, the mundane worker, the indifferent spouse or the misguided youth.

It is our time to become more relevant and more engaged in the world around us. To lead with our gifts and conscious intent, to feel the love and amazement of our neighbor and to seek a life of resilience against indifference and intolerance; this is worthy of personal commitment. We should be diligent in exercising our inner strength and liberate ourselves from people and situations that could do us harm, deem us irrelevant, make us vulnerable to the unguided objectives of others or keep us from a mindset focused on the vastness of our opportunity.

Awareness and growth however come at a price. To the immature or ignorant it may feel perfectly normal to avoid hardship and acquire knowledge, so they retreat and happily settle for the status quo. This kind of avoidance does not foster leadership, influence or economic increase. The opposite can be said for the unburdened and motivated as they do not shy away from their reality; they face trials with acquired knowledge, strength, character and humility. We can learn from them. They look for growth, opportunity and leadership, and are favored for their efforts. So let us ask ourselves, "What is my voice? What am I driven to accomplish in my life and am I on a harmonious path towards it? Through self-examination, what can I do right now to be proactive and redirect my efforts for better results? How can I better connect with the world around me by offering my gifts and talents, and how do I become authentic, relevant and masterful at it?" Simple, tell your story!

***

My story began in a hospital bed after my 5th cardiac event, this time it was a cardiac arrest; I died for 26 minutes. I was shocked with paddles 8 times, given 12 cardiac injections, and by all rights, I shouldn't even be here; but here I remain. A chain of events that I have no recollection of except for the sequence of events my doctors and family have told me. My wife found me lying motionless on our bed. She pulled me off, and performed CPR until two paramedic teams arrived. It was a horrific night for my family. Hospital physicians put me in an ice induced coma for two days and then slowly warmed me in order to reduce the risk of brain injury.

A pacemaker & defibrillator had been implanted in my chest as a safeguard against another cardiac arrest. As I woke from my coma, I was unaware of what had happened, but having spent my life in hospitals, I knew it was serious; I was completely vulnerable. I asked God if He was finished with me at the age of 50 and was today going to mark the extent of my mortality. But this wasn't a new thought, in actuality my story has been playing out for over 53 years. My heart has stopped and been shocked in over 30 separate events in my life, (8 of which occurred in my 4 open-heart surgeries, and another 8 during my cardiac arrest with the remainder as individual episodes), each one accompanied by this question: "Am I living my life to the potential God gave me, because there were 30 times he could have just let me go?"

How do I repay what I have been given and what have I mastered that could help someone else increase the value of their life, like mine has been? I decided to let God truly work through me, without strings and expectations, and this is what he decided upon: He wants me to teach the tools he has given me that allow us to make a difference in the world because of our character, our humility, our knowledge, our influence and our belief; how to be change agents for philanthropy in a global effort to mitigate poverty and burden, by being a force for abundance. So, here I am fulfilling this mission, and grateful for the opportunity.

This compact edition of my story does not illustrate my professional life, influence, brand or opportunities (which are required inclusions); it highlights only my critical path. This is just a sampling of the value and relate-ability I offer to my audiences.

Your story, your relate-ability, in whatever field of influence you purposely seek, can put you on the radar of, and sought after by, our global population. Your story, your platform of abundance and opportunity will help insulate you and those that follow or join you against social conformity and social oppression, which grow stronger each day. Be guarded against this false sense of security people get from conformity, it cannot be understated; it is one of the biggest enemies of entrepreneurship, and could make you and your purpose irrelevant. Challenge yourself to live at a higher personal standard and pare that philosophy to your mission. Students learn from their teachers because they are inspired to create and grow; everyone that hears your voice can become your student, understand that power and possibility. As you develop and grow your voice, always teach above your audience, because if they learn from you and acquire knowledge from you, they are more likely to follow and support you. However, in your quest to deliver your story, your mission, beware; if your story is too philosophical and unrelate-able you risk becoming irrelevant and without influence.

Everything that we consume becomes a part of who we are. This includes all of the useless junk, shallow entertainment, shock factors for the sake of ratings, stupidity and greed; all play a negative role in the efficacy of how others experience us. We need to be conscious of what we consume and emit, be mindful of the impressions and results we want to foster, as they will produce seedlings wherever they fall.

We all know people that hide behind ignorance, hoping for isolation from responsibility and risk, but in doing so they surrender their future; they believe it easier to disengage and let others shoulder their share of burden rather than stepping up to be counted, so they fall silent. Speak up, be the great director and producer of your own story, and deliver it in a compelling and meaningful fashion. Let your journey be experienced, don't sort out the challenges in order to mainstream or become competitive, and resist the urge to perform as an actor in order to gain appeal and support. Be masterful and intentional in your deliverance so that your message unfolds for your audience through your eyes. From this effort you become relate-able, worthy of time and consideration. Apprehension will surely surrender in order to make way for confidence and contribution, while simultaneously distancing you from conformity.

Too often we become like the aimless wanderer that side steps responsibility and reward only to let fear overshadow the power of conviction. Throughout the centuries leaders and monarchies were riddled with the non-committal, wills that were bent and often broken in order to conform, the individual silenced by the fear of success or never experienced the value that can be gained from a new idea, a different perspective…a point of view. The cascade effect from this apathy is present today. While prosperity reaches some, the mass indifference of a society towards poverty and struggle become the norm rather than the exception. These are some of the footprints that mark our history and that keep many of us from moving forward and being heard; but for those who step out from this path of rigidity, surrender the mundane lifestyle to become accountable and offer value free of expectation…..reward is granted.

Those of influence, (you) the 'Problem Solvers' can: change world politics, redirect an institutional norm to support the majority instead of the minority, provide understanding and opportunity where there is conflict, be the source of creative innovation for a fledgling endeavor, and be a teacher of abundance and economic prosperity. Beware; even great influence can fall to the dirt never reaching the magnitude it commands if it does not saddle a delivery system. The best form of leadership is to be 'seen' as-well-as 'heard'.

VISIBLE

> *Visible: devised to keep a particular part or item always in full view, readily seen or referred to.*

Influence and reach are best achieved through the use of a technological platform of education, creation and implementation. When you combine education with creation you achieve relate-ability, and when you combine creation with implementation you achieve transformation. Ultimately where relate-ability and transformation reside you find perpetual abundance. When you build your life and reach with this in mind, word of mouth about your excellent reputation and your servant leadership can expand your horizons and your influence beyond comprehension. However, be cognizant of the apathy that can surround your delivery platform.

Technology has made exponential strides in creating a more expressive and more productive society, but with that comes dependent complications. The mass habitual use of technology to satisfy appetites for reality shows that serves as entertainment crack, has steered us away from opportunities that fuel a greater purpose for influencing social change and economic increase. In order to achieve this we must embrace a life of courageous action and perpetual progress so that we remain visible and relevant.

No longer is it just goods and services that are sought after as commodities. We can leverage our talents, tools, resources and voice through a hosting platform, creating a new category of trade.

Be not afraid to be your own voice and face for change and increase. Be vulnerable and present yourself on a global platform with authenticity and humility, with focus on you, so that others can get to know you first and your cause second. Yes, be the face of your opportunity but don't let it overshadow your mission.

If your audience can relate with you they will look further. The mistake many make is they allow their objective, their job, their cause and their opportunity to be their mouth piece, which puts them at a disadvantage. Instead of learning about the value of the person presenting, the audience makes a decision about the efficacy and value of the offer, which can result in a message or mission unheard or overlooked simply because the sequence of introduction was incorrect.

As a society we identify through our responsibilities (our titles), and become subordinate to their agendas forgetting the most important of identities, our own. This holds us short of our influence and potential, so we must evolve and expose our independence; which is a key element in creating our brand. Unaware of how to do this we turn to mass conformity, marketing hype, outdated strategies and succumb to the overbearing voice of caution rather than exposing our character, our transparency and our humility. There is no better medium for this introduction than through self-promoted video, creating an electronic presence and brand for the global audience to experience. Video not only delivers our message, it captures our tone, our deliberateness, our passion, our conviction and our belief; through this we become relate-able and relevant to a similar audience with the goal of developing our 'tribe'.

Do not be afraid to memorialize your journey, hurdles and struggles, risks, losses & rewards, lessons and turning points that have guided you in life, this becomes your video story. By these admissions, you increase relevance. Your video will serve as your introduction to the global marketplace, but when coupled with your own personal website, your own home page hosting, you stand apart and become a strong contingent within your market space. This home page will become the hub where you link all of your causes, offerings and opportunities, both current and future. The best way for someone to connect with you, learn from you and join you is just to follow your name, so secure your name as your home page domain. Resist the motivation to develop a catchy title as your domain, this can become outdated and will only confuse your audience; however your name is timeless.

Overcoming a misconception: Your brand is not your company, your cause, your opportunity or what you pay a publicist to develop for you. Your brand is a set of public artifacts that reveal who you are, how you serve, and what people can expect from you in terms of image, value and service! Artifacts can be interviews, journals, videos, speeches, peer reviews, articles, etc... created by you or others about you. These are bits of information that help define you the person to those getting to know you. Display them on your site; give freely to your audience. If you don't currently have a library of these to choose from, make it a goal to go create them. With your brand, your image (when developed correctly), you are more likely to make it on the radar of the market audience you want to serve, and can increase the impact your mission deserves. Your brand, the value you offer will often solve problems others are searching through solutions for.

If you don't think that your brand, the impression you leave on someone through the application of your home page, is important above and beyond the company you represent, the cause you serve, the opportunity you offer, think again. Economists agree that 25% of the global populations are currently connected through web or cell phone platforms and that in 3-5 years that number will increase to 75%; that's an additional _3-billion_ new people. Your brand is both the best passive and active way to recruit to your mission. The recruiting masters, (the problem solvers) will capture the largest share of business and influence from this emerging group. In addition, infinite opportunities to partner with companies, influencers and causes to extend your reach and impact well beyond your own circles, await you. The recluse, the conformist and the riskless motion of the masses will choose to sidestep this process for sake of urgency and impatience. This avoidance does not foster leadership or economic increase. Resist the temptation to be subordinate to someone else's objective, become the problem solver to your market share and capture some of the _3-billion_.

Do not settle yourself to realistic goals; unlock the magnitude of your capability. Do not aim low; do not succumb to criticism from the conformists, for without commitment and will, ascension is out of reach.

Global struggles, individual challenges, lack of influence and declining individual economics provide the biggest opportunities, especially for the 'problem solvers'.

***

I look back at the joys in my life, celebrate and give thanks for my family, but I pay special attention to the challenges I faced because they are the ones that have held my feet to flame. I have never known life without cardiac challenges, and I will never escape that fact. I am grateful to be alive and able to create and contribute, but truth be known I am still a little scared of my mortality. With this admission comes clarity about how I live my day, the value I give, the transparent way I choose to do it, and the best way I can serve my God, my family and those with whom I have influence.

Are you living your life creating perpetual abundance to the magnitude you were born with, and is your 'story' being told?

"Each of us is born with phenomenal capacity to create and serve;

our choice throughout our life

is what we do with that knowledge."

WHAT ARE YOU DOING WITH YOURS?

"Sharing our truths can provide the opportunity for great healing."
~ Kristen Noel ~

Services Recommended by
The Wellness Fair

Your own personal story will help many people. Do you want to publish it in a book? If you're answer is yes, contact our publisher. They'll make it fast, easy, and affordable for you to get your story out of your head and into print!

Are you an accredited wellness professional?

Then you definitely need to publish a book. Think of the first six letters in the word authority? *USA Today* says 84% of people in the world want to write a book but far less than 1% actually do. Because of that, published authors are:

- Instant experts
- Instant authority figures
- Most trusted source of information
- Increased credibility
- Increased visibility
- ... and much, MUCH, more!

Imagine what that global perception will do for your business!

Authorpreneur Academy will not only make the writing and publishing process fun, quick, and easy, they'll train you on how to leverage your book to build your business before you even write one word!

Not a writer? Most entrepreneurs aren't! They offer a done-for-you service where you show up to just 7 phone calls and they take care of the rest, plus provide free training!

Because they don't work with just anyone, you first need to apply and be interviewed.

Start your book journey by applying today:
https://authorpreneur.academy/apply

"Keep taking time for yourself until you're you again."
~ Lalah Delia ~

Next Steps

There are many ways you can get involved with our community:

1. *Attend events* as a wellness enthusiasts

2. Consume our *wisdom sharing* materials

3. Be a *vendor* at a local trade fair nearest you

4. Once a vendor, you're able to be a *speaker*

5. Become a *co-author* in the next volume of this book series

6. Contribute to our *guest blog*

7. Contribute to our *quarterly magazine*

8. Be a *guest on our podcast*

9. *Volunteer* to make the events possible

10. *Sponsor* to help our community grow

11. *Get a license* to host events in your area

By partnering with us, you can leverage our community for an entire career; we'll train you how.

Does this seem like something you would be interested in?

Go to **www.TheWellnessFair.org** to join us today!

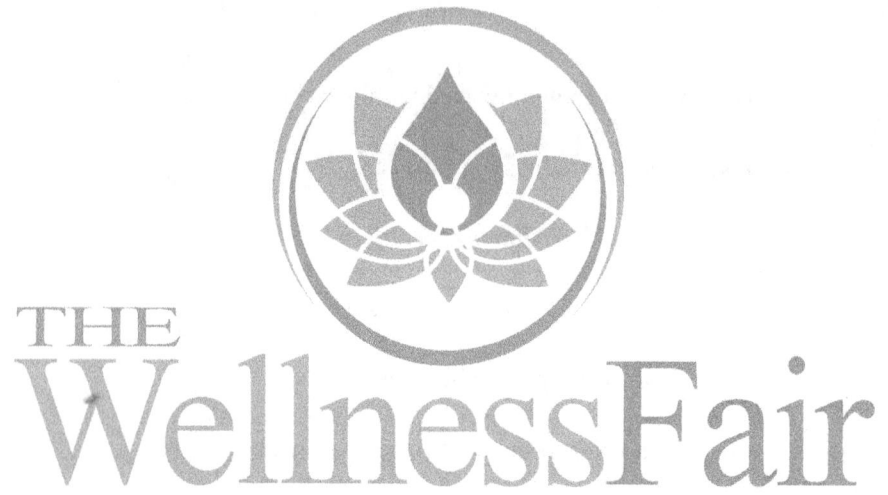

www.TheWellnessFair.org/2016Book